THE COMPLETE GUIDE TO NATUROPATHY

GALA

NATURE CURE
FOR COMMON DISEASES

By

Dr. Dhiren Gala

B.Sc., D.H.M.S., D.O., D.Ac.,
C.G.O., C.C.H., A.R.S.H.

Recipient of a gold medal for extraordinary
work in the field of Alternative Therapeutics

With

Dr. D. R. Gala

B.A.M.S., N.D., D.N.O., D.C.O.

Dr. Sanjay Gala

M.B. (BOM.), M.S. (ENT)

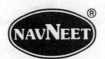

NAVNEET PUBLICATIONS (INDIA) LIMITED

Navneet House	Navneet Bhavan
Gurukul Road, Memnagar,	B. S. Road, Dadar,
Ahmadabad – 380 052.	Mumbai – 400 028.
Phone : 6630 5000	Phone : 6662 6565

DHANLAL BROTHERS DISTRIBUTORS

70, Princess Street, Mumbai – 400 002.
Phone : 2201 7027 / 2205 3716

G 4510

Visit us at : www.navneet.com | e-mail : npil@navneet.com

Price **$ 4.00**

Dr. D. R. Gala

1st floor, Abbas Building 'A',
Near Tilak Market, Jalbhai Lane,
Harkishandas Hospital Road,
Grant Road (East), Mumbai – 400 004.
Phone : 2386 7275
Timings : 4 to 7 p. m.

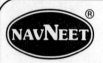 # NAVNEET PUBLICATIONS (INDIA) LIMITED

Mumbai : 1. Bhavani Shankar Road, Dadar, **Mumbai – 400 028.**
(Tel. 6662 6565 • Fax : 6662 6470)
2. **Navyug Distributors :** Road No. 8, M. I. D. C., Next to Indian Institute of Packaging, Marol, Andheri (East), **Mumbai – 400 093.**
(Tel. 2821 4186 • Fax : 2835 2758)

Ahmadabad : Navneet House, Gurukul Road, Memnagar, **Ahmadabad – 380 052.**
(Tel. 6630 5000)

Bengalore : Sri Balaji's, No. 12, 2nd Floor, 3rd Cross, Malleswaram, **Bengalore – 560 003.** (Tel. 2346 5740)

Chennai : 30, Sriram Nagar, North Street, Alwarpet, **Chennai – 600 018.**
(Tel. 2434 6404)

Delhi : 2-E/23, Orion Plaza, 2nd & 3rd Floor, Jhandewalan Extn., **New Delhi – 110 055.**
(Tel. 2361 0170)

Hyderabad : Kalki Plaza, Plot No. 67, Krishnapuri Colony, West Maredpalley, **Secunderabad – 500 026.** (Tel. 2780 0146)

Kolkata : 1st Floor, 7, Suren Tagore Road, **Kolkata – 700 019.** (Tel. 2460 4178)

Nagpur : 63, Opp. Shivaji Science College, Congress Nagar, **Nagpur – 440 012.**
(Tel. 242 1522)

Nashik : Dharmaraj Plaza, Old Gangapur Naka, Gangapur Road, **Nashik – 422 005.**
(Tel. 231 0627)

Navsari : 3/C, Arvind Nagar Society, Lunsikui Road, **Navsari – 396 445.** (Tel. 244 186)

Patna : 205, Jagdamba Tower, 2nd Floor, Sahdeo Mahto Marg, Srikrishnapuri, **Patna – 800 001.** (Tel. 254 0321)

Pune : Navneet Bhavan, 1302, Shukrawar Peth, Near Sanas Plaza, Bajirao Road, **Pune – 411 002.** (Tel. 2443 1007)

Surat : 1, Ground Floor, Sri Vallabh Complex, Kotwal Street, Nanpara, **Surat – 395 001.**
(Tel. 246 3927)

Vadodara : Near Hanuman Wadi, Sardar Bhuvan Khancho, **Vadodara – 390 001.**

PREFACE

People seem to be gradually losing faith in conventional therapeutic systems. Today, more and more people have come to entertain serious misgivings about all kinds of medication, and are now beginning to look upon Naturopathy as the ideal alternative to taking potions and nostrums.

A comprehensive survey carried out in the United Kingdom in 1970 showed that 90 per cent of the people had implicit faith in their family doctors, but within the span of only ten years, the situation changed drastically. A survey in 1980 revealed that the percentage of the population reposing complete faith in the family doctor fell short of even 40 per cent. This rapid erosion of faith is not only significant, but it also augurs well for the future of Naturopathy.

Some twenty years ago, it appeared that the battle against diseases was going to be won decisively with the help of the wonder drugs that were being discovered at that time. New and improved equipment and methods of diagnosis were being developed, and epidemics of infectious diseases were being brought under control one after another. The picture is not so rosy today. We are gradually becoming aware of the numerous side effects of drugs. If the drugs were really efficacious even the risk of side effects would have been over looked. But the reality is different. Despite the fact, that the expenditure incurred by the United States government on the protection and preservation of the health of its citizens is many times greater than that incurred by any other country, sad to say, more and more people there are falling victims to a wide variety of diseases, and a larger proportion of young lives are being lost than ever before.

It can, no longer, be denied that it is impossible to wipe out diseases merely by medication. What is necessary is that people should be inspired and encouraged to take an active interest in their own health, and to instruct them in the basic rules of the preservation of health. This is the principal aim of Naturopathy. Nature Cure does not employ the trial and error methods so prevalent today which are strikingly epitomised in the dictum : "If one medicine does not work, try another. If that one also fails, there is always a third one ..."

Naturopathy has a completely different approach to the treatment of diseases. Naturopathy defines disease as "disease", an absence of the feeling of well-being generated by robust health. Nature Cure does not attempt to get rid of illness, but aims primarily at restoring health. It does not attempt a frontal attack on the diseases or microbes, but endeavours to strengthen the natural defences of the body. In short, it is the body that effects the cure, not the physician.

It is doubtless true that people are turning, in ever increasing numbers, to Nature Cure, but many of them regard Nature Cure methods, fundamentally, in the same way as they regard other therapeutic systems, and try to evaluate the curative methods of Naturopathy by the standards of other systems. A single illustration will serve to explain this point. A person suffering from a chronic disease goes to a Naturopath, and is told that it would be necessary to fast for two to four days, and that for the next few days only simple uncooked food would have to be taken. At once the person exclaims, *"Why? my family doctor has always been telling me that one must take highly nutritious protein-rich food four times a day; otherwise one gets weakened, and the body gets emaciated, losing weight."* It is difficult to convince such a patient that the task of freeing the body from the disease, and that of maintaining its strength and weight, are different, and so the two cannot be accomplished simultaneously. If the patient keeps the medical counsel of the previous physician in mind and fasts, or restricts his diet, unwillingly, this negative attitude is bound to have an adverse effect on the body, resulting in weakness and slowing down of the rate of recovery. It is absolutely imperative that the patient adopts a method of treatment in full faith, and follows the prescribed regimen scrupulously.

Nature Cure methods have not yet become very popular in our country. People are still dazzled by the so-called wonder drugs and the huge sophisticated contraptions used for diagnosis. But as real understanding and education gain ascendance, the futility and dangers of drugs will become glaringly evident and the number of adherents of Naturopathy will surely increase manifold. The future of Naturopathy is, therefore, bright.

There is no room for doubt that if the reader studies, understands and practises the methods described in this book, he will be able to free himself from the threat of disease, and enjoy perfect health. Equipped with a mastery of Nature Cure methods, he will be able to treat and eliminate not only his own ailments, but also those of his near and dear ones.

In conclusion, we would gladly welcome from all our readers, any suggestions and opinions they would like to give about this book.

— *Authors*

CONTENTS

PART I : INTRODUCTION

1. Naturopathy or Naturism? 6
2. Why Naturopathy? 9
3. Must We Fall Ill? 19
4. History of Naturopathy 27
5. Principles of Naturopathy 34

PART II : THE TOOLS OF NATUROPATHY

6. Diet 43
7. Juice Diet 68
8. Fasting 70
9. Exercise 73
10. Hydrotherapy 92
11. Clay Therapy 108
12. Sun-Bath 111
13. Air-Bath 115
14. Massage 117
15. Magnetotherapy 120
16. Acupressure... 126

PART III : NATUROPATHY-IN PRACTICE

17. Nature Cure Treatments for Various Common
    Diseases (in Alphabetic Order) 130
18. Some Case Histories 165

□□□

PART I : INTRODUCTION

1. NATUROPATHY OR NATURISM?

Not many people are able to distinguish between living in accordance with the laws of Nature (Naturism, Nature Worship) and treatment of diseases in accordance with the laws of Nature (Naturopathy, Nature Cure). These two are not identical. It is important to understand the obvious as well as the subtle differences between these two ideologies.

The German physician Dr. Adolph Just and his followers can be regarded as the founders of Naturism, i.e., Nature Worship. Dr. Just's book 'Return to Nature' is the Bible of the proponents of Naturism. Their beliefs can be summarized as follows :

"Observe the animals in their natural habitat. Observe their daily routines, their ways of life. One generalization of universal applicability emerges from all such observations: all the animals obey the laws of Nature, and (as a consequence) enjoy excellent health. In return for obedience to the dictates of Nature, they have been generously endowed with good health by Nature. If at all there has been a failure to take advantage of this boon of Nature, the failure has been on the part of Man—the Lord of Creation! The reason is not that Man is odious to Mother Nature. Man is, in fact, the noblest creation of God, in His own image. He should be enjoying perfect health as a matter of course. Nevertheless, the fact remains that man is suffering from innumerable ailments. It has to be ruefully admitted that man himself is responsible for this sorry plight. While other animals follow and obey Nature, man perversely uses his intelligence in continually finding ways of transgressing Nature's laws and thus invites the calamity of ill health upon himself."

The proponents of Naturism exhort man to live in accordance with Nature's laws. In their opinion, all the ills of mankind can be traced to one single cause—Modern Civilization. There is only one solution for its problems—a Return to Nature. They advise us to reject all the appurtenances of civilization : from fire to television and radio, to eat only raw vegetarian food, live in the open, and lead a simple life.

This ideology found wide acceptance in Europe. In Germany, the Nature Worshippers went so far as to build large sanatoria where men and women of all ages led self-reliant lives, subsisting on vegetables and fruits, sleeping on the floor, communing with Nature and going about all their affairs in the nude. The cult became very popular in Germany. It was only in 1938, when Hitler compelled these adherents of Naturism to clothe themselves, that the world came to know that in Germany alone there were a million naked worshippers of Nature!

Now let us consider the ideology of the proponents of Nature Cure or Naturopathy.

While the proponents of Naturism believe in returning to Nature, the proponents of Nature Cure believe in advancing beyond Nature. The devotees of Naturism stop at worshipping Nature, but the adherents of Naturopathy endeavour to achieve a synthesis of such diverse but complementary elements as Nature and Art, Past and Future, or, in a nutshell, Nature and Civilization. They do not believe that the progress that civilization has achieved through the ages is without value; however, they do recommend the rejection of those elements of civilization which have proved detrimental, and even disastrous.

Thus, the proponents of Nature Cure concede the importance of Nature, but do not hesitate to assist Nature in combating diseases and to hasten the restoration of health by the adoption of extraneous curative measures like hydrotherapy, fasts, clay therapy, regulation of food, Magnetotherapy, Acupressure, etc.

Expert Naturopaths do not consider diagnosis of diseases superfluous. They carry out various tests and investigations to ascertain the causes of the disease and other relevant facts before prescribing treatment, thus ensuring that the treatment is rational, sound and appropriate. They also evaluate the progress of the process of recovery every few days. The treatment of common ailments is simple, but if there are complications, variations and refinements in the treatment may become necessary. If, in particular cases, they encounter limitations of Naturopathy, they do not hesitate to recommend alternative systems of medicine to the patient.

The main contention of this chapter is that though leading a completely natural life is, and should remain, our ideal, it is not wholly practicable in the present era, nor would it be reasonable to expect that the present-day industrial society will adopt an outmoded, 'stone age' way of life. Because people cannot lead their lives in complete consonance with the laws of Nature, they are inevitably going to suffer from major or minor ailments. They can be restored to health by adopting various Nature Cure measures like changes in their food habits, exercise, mud therapy, hydrotherapy etc. This system is simple, harmless and absolutely dependable, unlike most other systems.

It is possible for every individual to maintain his own health without recourse to professional assistance by adopting this system with an intelligent appreciation of the factors involved. Treatment of minor ailments can also be successfully undertaken by oneself. If we are careful about the maintenance of our health and keep a watchful eye on the state of health of our bodies, we shall not be compelled to run to the doctor for every minor disorder.

2. WHY NATUROPATHY ?

Is Naturopathy superior to other therapeutic systems ? Is it safer? These questions are bound to occur to anyone. Let us discuss them in detail.

Let us begin with a consideration of other systems. A majority of them rely on drugs for curing diseases. The devotees of drugs believe that drugs affect the body. This belief is erroneous, the reality being quite the contrary. **It is, in fact, the body that acts upon the drugs, and not the drugs upon the body.** This assertion may sound a little strange, but nonetheless it is true. There is a regulatory agency in the body that maintains its health. This agency is the "Vital force", the force that combats diseases. This Vital force acts continually, night and day, to preserve the health of the body. The moment a deleterious or unwholesome substance enters the body, the Vital force comes into play, concentrating on the task of ejecting the intrusive substance. For example, if a particle of dust lodges in the eye, there is an immediate and copious flow of tears. This flow has only one aim : to flush the particle out. Now, there is a large variety of remedial powders, called "surma", on the market in oriental countries. They are supposed to be beneficial for the eyes, allegedly by removing 'heat' from them. Application of such a powder in the eyes results immediately in a profuse flow of tears. The user is satisfied that the 'heat' of the eyes has been cast out. In point of fact, there has been no 'heat' cast out, nor any soothing coolness introduced. Nature has only been trying to wash the powder away in order to protect the eyes from the effects of the poisonous chemical (antimony) in the powder. It is not the 'surma' powder that acts on the eye, but the eye that acts on the powder. The same is the case with the various purgatives from the herbal preparation 'nepala' (croten), and countless other herbs, to milk of magnesia, consumed to relieve constipation. The Vital force endeavours to wash them out as quickly as possible to prevent them from harming the body.

Taking purgatives results not only in the elimination of waste products, but also in the discharge of a large quantity of water. Where has all this water come from? Obviously, it has been drawn from the blood. Just as the eyes secrete water in the form of tears in order to keep them clean, the inner lining of the intestines also secretes fluid to help the elimination of waste products. If this fluid (serum) is prodigally wasted, its secretion gradually diminishes. The habitual user of purgatives soon finds that the medicine no longer has the desired effect, unless the dosage is increased. A time comes when the desired effect cannot be obtained, no matter how large the dose that is taken. We say then that the body has become habituated or inured to the drug. The point is, if it is the medicine that acts on the body, how does it happen that a drug which induced motion of the bowels when taken in the normal dosage, fails, after a period of continued use, to have an effect even in much larger doses? In many cases of persons who have recklessly taken purgatives all their lives, it has been found during the course of operations or autopsies that their intestines had become as tough as horns. Just imagine what the intestines must have suffered, to lose their natural flexibility like that of the tongue, and become as tough and hard as horns!

Allopathic medicines very often induce adverse side effects. Even the widely used aspirin is not safe, according to Dr. James Roth, a professor at the Graduate School of Medicine, University of Pennsylvania, U.S.A. Dr. Roth's researches on the effects of various medicines on the digestive system have earned him worldwide recognition as an authority on these matters. *"Sixty to seventy per cent of the habitual users of aspirin eventually suffer from internal haemorrhage and anaemia,"* he warns. We are all aware of the side effects of penicillin, once considered a miracle drug. Thalidomide used to be looked upon as an innocuous sedative. But when women who had been taking the drug during pregnancy began to give births to babies with serious

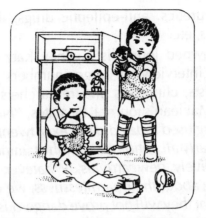

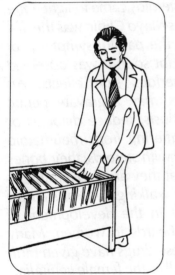
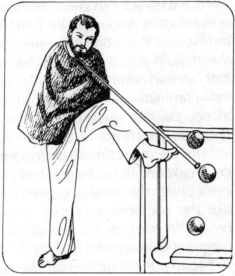

Fig. 2·1 : Thalidomide Tragedies

malformation of limbs – the 'Thalidomide babies' – it had to
be banned.

Do only aspirin, penicillin and thalidomide cause such
side effects? Are other drugs safe? It is not possible to answer
this sanguine question in the affirmative. The American
Medical Association has published a list of 72 drugs which
have serious side effects. The list includes sulpha drugs,
antibiotics, drugs used in the treatment of diabetes, sedatives,
sleeping pills, anti-rheumatic drugs, pain-killers, kidney

stimulants, diuretics, anti-epileptic drugs, thyroid extracts, anticoagulants, etc.

The renowned journalist Sydney Katz has written an article after interviewing large numbers of physicians, pharmacologists, clinicians and researchers. In the article, published in Maclean's journal, he states, *"Ninety per cent of the drugs being used today did not exist twenty or twenty-five years ago. Nearly all antibiotics, antihistamines and sedatives are comparatively new arrivals. Whatever the claims put forward today about their harmlessness, we cannot say with confidence that they will not prove dangerous in the future. In 1948, the miraculous effects of the steroids came to light. One of the doctors working at the famous Mayo Clinic was the first to discover that cortisone relieves the painful symptoms of rheumatoid arthritis immediately. But soon it was observed that steroid drugs can cause serious side effects. An indiscriminate use of these drugs may aggravate peptic ulcers, cause a relapse of tuberculosis, induce diabetes or bring on psychosis. If children suffering from rheumatoid arthritis are indiscriminately treated with steroids, their bones get weakened to such an extent that they are liable to break even under the stresses caused by walking. Use of steroids like the sex hormones may result in the development of breasts in men, or the growth of beards in women. Many pregnant women who had used these drugs have given birth to babies possessing the male as well as the female genitalia."*

Warning doctors against the indiscriminate use of steroids in the excessive enthusiasm of effecting cures overnight, Sydney Katz writes, *"It is absolutely necessary to exercise restraint in the treatment of diseases, and one must act on a war footing. If we do not take heed today, tomorrow's world will be populated by multitudes with defective hearts, damaged livers and kidneys and impaired visual, auditory and sexual functions, and by throngs of malformed babies."*

The Head of the Department of Pharmacology at the Bridham Hospital in Boston states unequivocally, *"No drug can be considered safe."*

Another shortcoming of traditional therapeutics is the tendency to treat each symptom of a disease individually. Dr. William Gutman of New York Medical College states, *"This system treats each symptom in isolation, prescribing analgesics for pain, antipyretics for fever, laxatives for constipation, etc."*

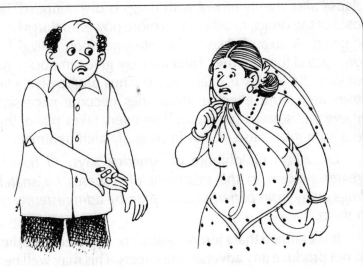

Wife   : (to sick husband returning from a visit to the doctor) : What a lot of tablets! Must you take so many?

Husband : Yes. These yellow tablets are for the liver, these green ones for the stomach, and the white ones for the kidneys.

Wife   : And the red ones?

Husband : The doctor did not say anything about them. But perhaps they are intended to regulate the traffic of the other tablets.

Fig. 2·2 : The Terrific Tale of Tablets

Dr. Gutman goes on to state, *"This means that the system does not take an overall, integrated view of the patient and the illness. Medicines may be useful as palliatives till the Vital force becomes activated, but their usefulness ends there. Actually, if the Vital force has been weakened beyond repair, medicines are of no avail."*

If efforts are aimed only at symptomatic relief, the disease itself is lost sight of. Such attempts can admittedly suppress the disease, but create fresh problems later on.

Another important aspect of the matter is that treatment of each symptom separately necessitates large doses of medicines; this is a great drawback in itself. In case there is a relapse after the treatment with drugs is discontinued, larger doses of the drugs, or other even more powerful drugs have to be given. A laxative leaves the intestines more sluggish and constipated than before. Antacids may give temporary relief, but later the acidity is exacerbated. Thus progressively larger doses and more effective medicines become necessary to relieve the isolated symptom. If recovery takes place, then it does so not because of, but in spite of, such treatment.

Dr. Alton Goldbloom of America says, *"I have had greater success in the treatment of diseases by snatching drugs away from patients rather than by administering drugs to them."*

It is claimed that Homoeopathic or Ayurvedic medicines do not produce any adverse side effects. This may well be true to a certain extent. But no practitioner of these systems can deny that the administration of one medicine in place of another, or excessive doses, can be harmful. And cases of erroneous prescriptions or dosages are more frequent than we imagine. There is also the appalling problem of adulteration. Only recently a number of deaths were caused by adulterated medicines in the reputed government-run hospital in Bombay, the J. J. Hospital. Wouldn't a therapeutic system effecting cures without the use of any medication be a much more logical choice?

Two other points deserve careful consideration. With the sole exception of Ayurveda, the indigenous Indian system of medicine, the history of rational therapeutics is not very old. In particular, the supposedly infallible medicines of Allopathy have come into existence only very recently. Does this mean that there were no cures before that ? Did every major or

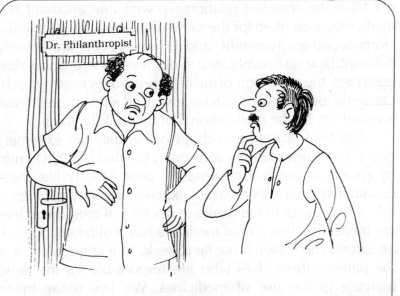

The doctor had assured me that he would set me on my feet in two months. And he has kept his word; I have had to sell my car to pay his bills.

Fig. 2·3 : Cost of Medication

minor illness inevitably end in death ? The answer to this question is obvious: Cures have been effected from time immemorial. Doctors have had no difficulty through the ages in maintaining their exalted status in society.

Records show that at various periods in history, cures have been effected by administering excreta of animals, powdered corpses, saw-dust, saliva and blood of lizards, dried and pulverized snakes, semen of frogs, crabs' eyes, roots of herbs, horns and fat of animals, etc. Now, if diseases have been cured by what we would regard today as quack remedies, there can be only one explanation: the cures were effected not by the medicines, but by the reactivation of the Vital force, in spite of the administration of such grotesque medicines.

Another point to be considered is this : How can the same disease be cured by many different medicines which do not have the remotest relationship with one another ? The medicines prescribed for the same disease by the Allopathic, Homoeopathic, Ayurvedic and Unani systems are entirely different, bear no resemblance to one another in any way; but even then, the symptoms of the disease are alleviated by each. Only one logical reason can be advanced for this: the disease is cured not by the medication, but by the Vital force.

The final objection to drugs is that they are extremely costly. Every one of us has seen many families brought to ruin by enormous medical expenses. A poor country like India cannot afford such extravagant expenditure on medicines.

It may occur to the reader to ask why, if most medicines are ineffective, this cult of medicine has proliferated to such an extent. The reason is not far to seek. To a large extent, it is the patients themselves who are responsible for the rapid increase in the use of medicines. We live today in an "instant" civilisation. We have come to expect instant service, instant food, instant results. We also insist on instant relief from sickness or pain. If a person is depressed, he wants an instant lift (pep pills). If he is tired, he wants instant rest (a tranquiliser or sleeping pill). If he has an infection, he wants an instant cure (antibiotics). The current slogan is : 'Do something *now'*. The drug industry and the medical practitioners know this, and, as a result, are making hay. We lose sight of the fact that illness is the result of a long period of violations of Nature's laws, such as indulgence in unwholesome foods and habits. Consequently, a cure also would naturally require a reasonable period. The average man is not at all prepared to change his life-style to maintain or regain health. He keeps on inviting illness by transgressing every rule of health. When the illness strikes, he goes to extreme lengths to suppress the disease by the use of medicines. A majority of doctors will testify that people have no real desire for health. When they fall ill, all they want to do is to patch up their health by suppressing the symptoms. As soon as they obtain some relief, they go back to their old ways and indulge in excesses.

We have already emphasised the fact that no disease is created overnight. A disease that manifests itself today has been developing for a long time. It is natural that a cure will also take some significant time. However, Naturopathy takes less time to effect a cure than people imagine. Cold, cough, influenza, fever, boils and such other complaints are cured by fasting for only a few days. Even chronic illnesses can be got rid of quickly enough by adopting an integrated plan of fasting, changes of diet, exercise, hydrotherapy and other Nature Cure remedial procedures. A friend of mine, an extremely busy practitioner of Homoeopathy, undertakes the treatment of a patient only after stipulating that the patient will continue his treatment for at least three months. People are known to have kept on taking medicine for six months, nine months, or even longer. Why should Nature Cure methods be then charged with being unduly dilatory?

It is the misfortune of the Nature Cure system that people adopt it as the very last resort after having tried all other systems, and in the process, having reduced their bodies to wrecks and having extinguished the flame of the Vital force by the use of a large variety of drugs – and despite all this, they expect Nature Cure to provide them with instant cure. And it is the good fortune of such people that Naturopathy does not disappoint them, but free them from diseases, often sooner than expected.

Every Nature Cure measure has only one aim: to strengthen the natural resistance of the body to diseases, i.e., to activate the Vital force, and to get rid of the poisons accumulated in the body. A cure effected by Nature Cure methods is a sign of the Vital force having been strengthened. This is proved by the fact that once a cure has been effected by these methods, no other illness attacks the person for a long time.

Nature Cure induces people to take an active interest in their health. A patient going to a physician for medicines has to remain a mute spectator, but in Nature Cure, the patient is required to play the main role, and so has necessarily to critically analyze his illness, his dietary habits, his way of life, etc. Thus he gets involved in the process. It is an incontrovertible fact that, if the patient is actively interested in the causes and the treatment of his illness, the illness must speedily take to flight. The way the famous American journalist Norman Cousins freed himself from an incurable disease like Ankylosing Spondylosis is a striking example.*

In summarising this chapter, it can be said that Nature Cure is a unique science with an unlimited potentiality to cure almost all diseases. With the exception of a few diseases which require surgical intervention, all diseases can be tamed by Nature Cure and made as docile as the proverbial cow. This system not only removes the symptoms, but also exterminates the disease. It strikes at the very root of the disease. It shows man the right way to a healthy life, and inculcates the virtues of discipline and self-control. Moreover, it entails little expense. It will be no exaggeration to say that Nature Cure will become the principal therapeutic system of the twenty-first century.

––––––––––––

* For a thrilling and instructive account of the victory of Norman Cousins over the disease, read the book 'Anatomy of an illness' W.W. Norton and Co. Inc., New York.

3. MUST WE FALL ILL?

"Prevention is better than cure." In other words, "Don't ever fall ill."

The moment you are given this advice, you are sure to retort, "But who wants to fall ill at all? Do you think it is up to us to decide whether to fall ill or not?"

The answer is : Yes, it is. It is entirely within the power of every one of us to maintain health and avoid falling a prey to illnesses.

There is a regulatory agency in the human body that protects it against diseases. This agency is termed the Vital force. If not seriously interfered with, the Vital force is capable of keeping the body free from illness all one's life. This means that, if care is taken to maintain the Vital force at its full strength, no disease can invade the body. And even if, due to some mischance, one does happen to be victimised by illness, it is certain that the illness will be speedily cast out by the Vital force. It is significant that even Hippocrates, the father of modern therapeutic science, believed that *"It is Nature that heals, not the physician."*

In order to be able to prevent illness, it is necessary to understand the factors that are responsible for weakening the Vital force. The following factors enfeeble the Vital force and cause the accumulation of poisons in the body :

(1) **Improper Dietary Habits :** Our ancestors lived on a very simple diet. It was precisely because of this that they enjoyed long lives. On the other hand, our food today abounds in spicy, fried preparations, cold dishes and sweets. The use of refined, processed and frozen foods is spreading. These foods produce large amounts of acidic and poisonous end-products in the body. Poisons accumulate even faster in the bodies of persons given to eating meat, or large amounts of pulses. And it is these poisons that are the roots of all disorders.

It is also necessary to think of the ingredients of the foods. Our food is made up of three chief ingredients : proteins, fats, and carbohydrates. Carbohydrates are digested partly in the mouth while chewing, and partly in the small intestine. Proteins are digested in the stomach, while fats are digested in the intestines. The digestion of each of these ingredients of food is a different, independent process. Now, if all the three ingredients are taken in large quantities in a single meal, they cannot be digested properly. The food will, in such cases, decay in the intestines and produce toxic substances.

The composition and compatibility of different foods are discussed in greater detail in chapter 6.

In addition to the quality, the kind and the make-up of the food, it is also necessary to think of its quantity. Today people do not exercise discretion in the amount of food they take. Food these days is so spicy and savoury that the temptation to eat more– and then just a little more!– cannot be easily resisted.

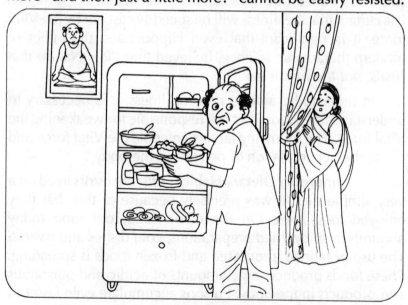

Fig. 3·1

Moreover, in our society, regaling people with food is considered a token of affection. We, therefore, stuff our guests full, urging them to eat more and more. Excessive amounts of food are a burden on the digestive system, and disrupt the process of digestion. Frequent feeds have the same effect. Burdening the digestive organs with more food before the digestion of one meal is completed, is senseless. The words of that master of health science, Redi Mallet, deserve to be carved in our dining halls : *To keep healthy, one must always remain a little hungry.*

The use of sugar and salt has also increased enormously. All the experts are unanimous in denouncing both of these substances as deleterious. Sugar – and foodstuffs – containing substantial amounts of sugar, such as chocolate, peppermint,

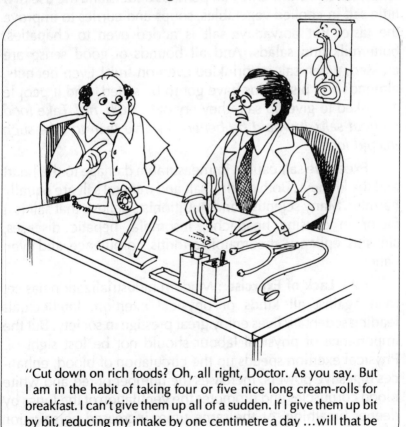

"Cut down on rich foods? Oh, all right, Doctor. As you say. But I am in the habit of taking four or five nice long cream-rolls for breakfast. I can't give them up all of a sudden. If I give them up bit by bit, reducing my intake by one centimetre a day ...will that be all right?"

Fig. 3·2

chewing gum, jams, jellies, sweets and foods canned in syrup–when taken in excess, cause tooth decay, diabetes, heart disease, migraine, skin eruptions and kidney disorders. This is why nutritionists have dubbed sugar 'sweet poison'. The famous British scientist Prof. John Yudkin, after numerous investigations, came to the conclusion that the human body needs no refined sugar as fuel for energy. The requisite amount of sugar is available in sufficient quantities from natural foods.

The use of salt too, like that of sugar, has exceeded all reasonable bounds. One can perhaps understand the use of a little salt in cooked vegetables, soups and curries to improve the taste. But nowadays salt is added even to chapaties, buttermilk and salads. And all bounds of good sense are crossed, when salt is sprinkled even on fruit! Even peanuts, almonds and pistachios have got to be salted. And, if people are asked to give up salt, they cry out : *"Oh, no! Take food without salt? It would be better to starve than to take such insipid food."*

Excessive salt causes immeasurable damage to the heart and the kidneys. Both marine salt and mineral salt are equally harmful. Many scientists and nutritionists believe that salt is a factor in causing headache, insomnia, hepatic diseases, sinusitis, epilepsy, rheumatoid arthritis, corpulence, and even cancer.

(2) **Lack of Exercise :** Modern industrialization has set man against all kinds of physical exertion. Intellectuals leading sedentary lives enjoy great prestige in society. But the importance of physical labour should not be lost sight of. Physical exertion speeds up the circulation of blood, enhances digestive powers, increases the number of red and white blood corpuscles and promotes the ventilation of the lungs by deeper breathing. At the same time, increased perspiration helps to remove some of the poisons from the body.

People leading sedentary lives cannot digest their food well. They are always suffering from indigestion, flatulence and constipation. And, as everyone knows, constipation is the mother of a host of disorders.

(3) **Irregular Life-style** : The numerous pressures of the business of making a living compel modern man to continually run hither and thither, as exigencies demand. As a result, he finds it impossible to live a regular life : taking his food, drinks and rest as and when he can, instead of following a regular schedule. The biological rhythm is consequently disrupted. He does not feel hungry when he should; the bowels do not move at the proper time; the intestines fill with toxic wastes; the body loses animation and is overcome by lassitude. This situation invites various diseases.

(4) **Addiction** : These days people accord high priority to sensual pleasures, and therefore become easy preys to objectionable and harmful habits such as addiction to stimulants like tea, coffee or cocoa, or intoxicants like tobacco, alcohol and drugs. We promote the formation and accumulation of toxic substances in the body by the consumption of such intoxicants, and invite dreadful diseases like cancer by keeping our mouths stuffed with betel leaves laced with tobacco, tobacco extracts, and even worse additives.

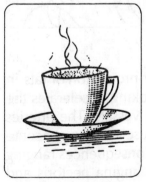

Fig. 3·3

Tea, coffee and cocoa are classified as stimulants. They contain caffeine and tannin, both of which are harmful substances. They affect specific parts of the brain, thus stimulating nerves and muscles, causing palpitations and quickened breathing. Coffee increases the proportion of fats in the blood. If this condition persists for a long time, the fat gets deposited on the walls of the blood vessels which get hardened and constricted. Gradually the blood pressure rises, the heart is overburdened, and the risk of a heart attack increases.

None of the beverages mentioned above possesses any

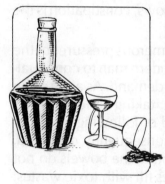

Fig. 3·4

nutritive value. The consumption of these beverages must be avoided.

Alcoholic drinks too, like tea and coffee, have deleterious effects on the nerves and the heart. Their effects on the digestive system are also well known. Alcohol blunts hunger, causes irritation and swelling of the lining of the stomach, and impairs the functions of the liver. These facts point clearly to the necessity of giving up, and abstaining from, the use of all types of alcoholic drinks.

The direct relation between smoking and heart disease has been established beyond doubt. Tobacco contains nicotine, which is explicitly described in medical dictionaries as a powerful and active poison. Smoking introduces this poison, as well as the highly poisonous gas carbon monoxide, into the lungs.

Experiments have shown that nicotine causes increased secretion of adrenalin and noradrenalin into the

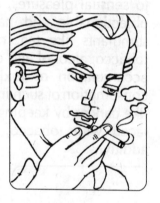

Fig. 3.5

blood stream, which results in a higher proportion of fats in the blood. It is for this reason that smoking accelerates the process of the hardening of the blood vessels. The arteries providing nutrients to the heart muscles also become congested, hardened and brittle, with consequences ranging from palpitations and hypertension to angina pectoris and heart attacks.

Vitamins are essential for the heart and the blood vessels. Vitamins stored in the body are gradually destroyed by smoking. Smoking just one cigarette destroys an amount of vitamin C equivalent to that contained in one whole orange.

Prolonged use of tobacco gives rise to palsy, vertigo, fainting fits and other nervous disorders. Sixteen carcinogens have been found to be present in tobacco. Long-term users of tobacco suffer from 'Buerger's Disease', in which the veins of the legs are constricted to such an extent that walking even a short distance causes excruciating pains in the calves.

And we should not run away with the idea that it is only smoking tobacco that harms the heart and impairs general bodily health. Chewing tobacco, applying tobacco powder or paste to the teeth and inhaling snuff are also harmful, to a smaller or a greater extent.

All packets of cigarettes bear the warning that cigarette smoking is injurious to health. In spite of this ubiquitous warning, not only the illiterate who have the excuse of not being able to read the warning, but even the literate find it impossible to give up smoking, once they have fallen victims to the habit. A recent survey revealed that nearly 80 per cent of doctors– yes, doctors– are addicted to smoking! This surely is the climax of man's slavery to the habit.

(5) **Psychological Factors :** In today's bustling and competitive life, mental tension has exceeded all bounds. Today we find countless people with a negative approach to life. It is a fact that mental attitude has a direct effect on the body. In the opinion of experts, a major proportion of the disorders of mankind are psychosomatic.

(6) **Indiscriminate Use of Medicines :** A large number of medicines are toxic in nature, and their use results in the accumulation of poisons in the body. They inactivate the bone marrow, thus weakening the Vital force. Obviously, when the Vital force itself is moribund, no medicines are going to be effective.

In the opinion of Dr. H. P. Pickeril, M. D., *"The only logical way to fight disease is to augment the power of the patient's body to resist diseases."*

According to Dr. Wendell McLeod, the Head of the Department of Medicine at the Saskechevan University of

Canada, *"It is most regrettable that we are bent upon making ever increasing use of medicines, instead of relying on, and having faith in, Nature's powers of resistance to diseases."*

Dr. H. G. Cox, M. D., of the New York College of Physicians and Surgeons, admonishes doctors in these words, *"The fewer the medicines you give to your patients, the better for them."*

The following words of the great pharmacologist and physician, Dr. William Osler, whose name is recorded in golden letters in history, deserve to be inscribed in the hearts of every one of us : *"The human body is such a complex machine that our present knowledge of it can still be considered only rudimentary. And yet we fill it with medicines about the mode of action of which we know next to nothing. The only real doctor is one who understands the limitations of his own medicines."* Perhaps no one is more qualified than Dr. Osler to express an opinion on the value of medicines.

The above dicta may perhaps seem unfounded, and even biased, to those doctors who are dazzled by the progress of medical science, and regard mechanistic therapeutic systems with admiration. But it is the opinion of Dr. Otto Mosset that, *"Science can hold only the second place to Nature's first. Notwithstanding all the progress that we have made in chemistry, it is not possible for all the laboratories in the world, uniting in a concerted effort, to equal the fine coordination and precision of the reactions continually occurring in every single cell of the body."*

The great inventor Thomas Alva Edison has very aptly remarked, *"So long as man is unable to produce even a blade of grass from non-living matter, Nature can continue to laugh at his vaunted scientific knowledge."*

----

4. HISTORY OF NATUROPATHY

Naturopathy is not of recent origin. It can be said to have originated 2500 years ago, at the time of Hippocrates. People regard Hippocrates as the father of modern medical science. This is a misconception. As a matter of fact, he owes his fame primarily to his advocacy of methods of healing based on the laws of Nature. Physis means Nature. It is from this Greek word that the term physician has been derived. He was the first to study the process of what has been described as 'healing crisis': the process that is the backbone of the Nature Cure system. It is this process that is described by Drug Therapists as the 'acute' state of a disease.

But the movement for the promotion of modern Naturopathy got under way some 150 years ago. The credit for this goes to Dr. Vincenz Priesnitz. He established a sanatorium at Grafenburg in Germany. Priesnitz himself suffered from ill-health for years. This man, endowed with perspicacity and insight, carried out investigations on the healing powers of cold water. Having regained his health by the use of cold baths, he went on to treat numerous patients successfully by hydrotherapy.

Priesnitz's successes with hydrotherapy spread his fame far and wide. People from far off places began to flock to him. His sanatorium became a place of pilgrimage for ardent devotees of health. His golden success was a thorn in the side of the practitioners of traditional systems of medicine. Like all innovators, Priesnitz had to face vigorous opposition from the conservative sections of society, which pelted him with libels, ridicule and abuses, and invoked the sanctions of the law against him. But truth triumphed in the end. This vicious persecution, and his success in overcoming it, served only to add to his prestige and reputation. Thus his opponents themselves became instrumental in spreading his fame.

His experiences had led Dr. Priesnitz to the firm belief that the cause of disease lies solely in the accumulation of poisons in the body as a result of a wrong way of life. If the natural defences of the body are strengthened, diseases disappear spontaneously. In his opinion, diseases do not come into existence overnight, but are the results of gradual accumulation of toxic substances in the body over long periods of time. The process of healing, as a consequence, must inevitably be somewhat slow. It is necessary to continue treatment with diligence and patience. A plaque bearing the legend 'YOU WILL HAVE TO BE PATIENT', placed near the entrance of Dr. Priesnitz's sanatorium, was intended to convey this truth. Dr. Priesnitz's views remain unchallenged even today.

Around that time an Austrian physician, Dr. Johannes Schroth, established another sanatorium in Liendweiz, a village in Czechoslovakia. Initially, he used to treat dogs, horses and cattle. Success in treating them encouraged him to undertake treatment of humans too. His fame began to spread with each success in treatment. But jealousy reared its ugly head once again, subjecting Dr. Schroth to the same harassment and persecution that Dr. Priesnitz had suffered. Contemporary doctors left no stone unturned in opposing him. Dr. Schroth struggled against hatred and insults for twenty years, and even suffered imprisonment. But his fortunes took a turn for the better in 1846, as a result of a singular occurrence. The Duke of Wintumburg was injured in the leg. The wound, deemed trivial at the time, soon assumed a dangerous aspect. Treatment by prominent doctors proved of no avail, and the Duke was ultimately advised to have the leg amputated, failing which, the doctors feared, the life of the Duke would be endangered. The Duke trembled at the very thought of living for the rest of his life as a cripple. The conviction that death could be no worse than a life of dependence brought him to Johannes Schroth's door, as a last resort. Schroth comforted him and began treatment. In a few months, the Duke recovered completely.

This event caused a sensation in the whole country. Schroth's critics were silenced. The Duke published an account of his treatment in a booklet, which was distributed to the people. Schroth's system of healing came to be recognised as valid by a large number of doctors, and some of them even embarked on a study of the system. There still were some critics of the system, but their criticism had lost its sting. While Priesnitz had demonstrated the therapeutic value of cold water, Schroth gave pride of place to treatment with hot and cold compresses, and fomentation. He also stressed the importance of dietetics.

Some time later, Father Sebastian Kneipp of Baveria (in Germany) attained fame as a healer. He was not only a Naturopath, but also a teacher and a social worker. He ran a sanatorium based on hydrotherapy for more than forty-five years, and attained exemplary success in curing all types of diseases. His book on hydrotherapy, 'My Water Cure', is studied with interest even today. His speciality was the use of water at different temperatures for different illnesses.

Among the outstanding healers of the last century was Dr. Arnold Rickley. He established the importance of air and sunlight in addition to water and diet. He believed constipation to be the root of all disorders, and gave top priority to its treatment. He himself was a strict vegetarian. Despite a childhood ridden with various ailments, the robust health he gained and maintained in his later life made him a living proof of the efficacy of Nature Cure. He attained the ripe old age of 97 years.

The contribution of Dr. Heinrich Lahmann of Germany to the development of Nature Cure is also of considerable importance. In his clinic in Dresden, treatment was based mainly on diet. Dietetics will remain indebted to him for his investigations in various areas like the quality and composition of diet that was required for maintenance of health, the deleterious effects of salt, and the havoc caused by addiction to intoxicants like alcohol.

Probably, the greatest exponent of Nature Cure was the German physician Dr. Louis Kuhne. At the comparatively tender age of twenty, his health had been completely ruined. After years of trying various medicines without success, he turned to Nature Cure as a drowning man clutches at a straw. Speedy and almost miraculous recovery made him an ardent supporter of Nature Cure. He studied Naturopathy, and established a health resort at Leipzig in 1886. His methods of treatment included sun-baths, steam-baths, hip-baths, etc. According to Kuhne, cleanliness of the body and purity of the blood were the only answers to diseases. He was the discoverer of the system of diagnosis based on the examination of the face and the neck. His books, 'The New Science of Healing' and 'The Science of Facial Expression', brought him universal recognition. The former book has been translated into nearly all the languages of the world. Louis Kuhne held that **"All diseases originate in the accumulation of poisons in the body; all diseases are fundamentally the same."** This principle has come to be accepted as the cornerstone of modern Naturopathy.

Another German adherent of Nature Cure, Dr. Adolf Just, is also considered an eminent Naturopath. He established a health home, 'Jungban', in the Herz Mountains. He discovered the method of healing with the help of clay, or mud. He was a firm believer in living in complete harmony with Nature. His book 'Return to Nature' became immensely popular. He proved that, by following the ancient natural life-style of mankind, and rejecting all artificial appurtenances of the supposedly civilized modern life, it is possible for one to regenerate and rejuvenate oneself. He was a staunch opponent of vaccination.

America also has made great contributions to the development of Naturopathy. In America the movement was led by Dr. James C. Jackson. At the age of 35 he became the victim of a serious disorder, which was declared to be incurable by physicians. After trying all sorts of remedies, with disappointing results, he turned to Dr. Silas Gleason, a disciple of Dr. Vincenz Priesnitz. Once more Nature Cure treatment demonstrated its superiority, and yielded gratifying results. Now Jackson was no longer merely a patient of Dr. Gleason, but joined him as his co-worker. At the same time he secured admission to the medical college there, eventually taking his degree in medicine and obtaining a licence to practise as a physician. He then set up the Jackson Sanatorium in Dansville, New York. He dispensed with the use of medicines, preferring to heal by Nature Cure methods, including hydrotherapy, systematic exercises, diet, psychological rehabilitation, rest, etc.

Another American exponent of Nature Cure to achieve eminence was Dr. Russell Trall. Despite his training in traditional therapeutics in a medical college, he resorted to Nature Cure methods in his later life. He founded the Hygienic Therapeutic College at Florence, New York. He authored numerous works on Naturism and Naturopathy.

Equally eminent as a Naturopath is Dr. J. H. Kellogg, the Director of the world-famous 'Battle Creek Sanatorium', Michigan State, U.S.A. Dr. Kellogg, an ardent supporter of hydropathy, sun-bathing, physiotherapy, etc., has written a number of books on these subjects.

Dr. Henry Lindlahr is another American Naturopath of renown. He exerted a decisive influence on the philosophy and methods of the Nature Cure System. He put forward the principle that every **acute disease was merely the sign of, or the manifestation of, the healing powers of Nature.** This principle has become one of the basic tenets of the Nature Cure therapeutic system. He did exemplary work in correlating the various aspects of Naturopathy and perfecting it as a unified scientific system. He was a firm believer in Iris Diagnosis. Two of his books, 'Iridiagnosis' and 'The Philosophy and Practice of Natural Therapeutics' have become widely known as authoritative works. Before adopting Nature Cure, he was a practitioner of Allopathy. But he realized the futility of traditional medicine during the course of the treatment of one of his own ailments. This gave a new turn to his life. He discarded all medicines, and all remedies relying on medicines. Initially, he resorted to Nature Cure methods for the treatment of his own ailment, and then went on to achieve fame as a great Naturopath.

Perhaps the greatest exponent of Nature Cure in the United States was Dr. J. H. Tilden. He established that, if one gives up harmful habits and erroneous ways of life, and adopts a proper life-style, good health is the inevitable result. Mend your habits, and cure follows. He was a great thinker and a distinguished author. 'Impaired Health' is his most well-known work.

Dr. Bernarr McFadden, a highly competent and popular exponent of Nature Cure, achieved great eminence, his fame spreading to the ends of the earth. He was an enthusiastic proponent of fasting, milk (lacto-) therapy and physical culture. His great work, 'The Encyclopaedia of Health', is the most comprehensive reference book in this field, in which every aspect of Nature Cure is discussed authoritatively, and in depth.

No history of Naturopathy would be complete without the mention of Dr. Benedict Lust, a disciple of Father Kneipp, and a staunch proponent of Juice Therapy.

Dr. Dewey, Dr. McCane (the famous dietician), Dr. Still (the father of Osteopathy), Dr. Daniel Palmer (the originator of the Cheiropractic System) also must receive honourable mention. Others like Dr. Bilz, Dr. Otto Jutner, Dr. Wigmore, etc. have worked hard to popularise Nature Cure.

In our country, too, great contributions to this system have been made by some mighty proponents. Among them are Mahatma Gandhi, Mr. Morarji Desai, Dr. Dinshaw Mehta, Dr. Lakshman Sharma, Dr. Janaki Sharan Varma, Dr. Kul Ranjan Mukherjee, Dr. Vitthaldas Modi, Dr. J. M. Jassawala, Dr. M. M. Bhamagara, Dr. S. J. Singh, Dr. Ramanlal Engineer, Dr. Krishna Varma, Dr. Shankarbhai Dave and Dr. Bhupatray Dave.

Magnetotherapy, Acupuncture, Acupressure, Yoga Therapy, Chromotherapy and other similar systems can be considered to be the parts of the Nature Cure system of therapeutics. It can be confidently asserted that because of the co-ordination and incorporation of all these systems, Nature Cure today has become capable of achieving quicker and lasting cures.

5. PRINCIPLES OF NATUROPATHY

'The Principle of the Unity of the Causes of Diseases' is the first basic principle of Naturopathy.

According to this principle, **there is one and only one cause of all diseases : the accumulation of toxic and foreign substances in the body, i.e., toxaemia.**

There are many contributory causes of such accumulation. Our body is made up of myriads of cells. Large numbers of these cells die, and are replaced by new cells, every day. The dead cells are foreign materials to the body. In addition, some processes in the living cells also continually form toxic wastes because of the metabolic reactions taking place in them. But the prime cause of the accumulation of poisons is the artificiality of our ways of life. Wrong, improper or misguided ways of life cause the production of large amounts of toxic substances in the body. If these poisons are not eliminated at reasonably fast rates, they accumulate in the body, resulting ultimately in a diseased condition. Thus, to a large extent, we ourselves are responsible for the accumulation of poisons in our bodies.

The efforts of the body to get rid of these poisons produce fever, swelling, pain and various other symptoms. When the effects of these attempts become noticeable in a particular part of the body, that organ or part of the body is regarded as diseased. In fact, **acute disease is merely a manifestation of the natural healing processes in the body.** We may choose to give various names to diseases, but it is clear that no matter what the disease is, and which part of the body it seems to affect basically, there is only one root cause : the accumulation of poisons in the body.

Thus, the sole cause of disease is the accumulation of poisons in the body. What we deem to be the symptoms of the disease are merely the outward manifestations of the natural efforts of the body to cast out the poisons.

Modern medical science attributes the causation of diseases to bacteria, viruses, fungi and other micro-organisms. And as a result of persistent propaganda most people have come to accept this as a fact. But it is a totally erroneous belief. Perhaps it would not be out of place to elaborate this important point here.

There are two kinds of micro-organisms : (1) Saprophytic micro-organisms that live on dead or non-living organic matter, and (2) Parasitic micro-organisms that live on nutrients obtained from living animals or plants.

Ninety-eight per cent of the micro-organisms on the earth have been classified as saphrophytic. They can be regarded as the sweepers and cleaners of Nature. They transform dead organic matter in the soil into substances that are essential for the growth of plants. And plants are directly or indirectly the main source of nutrients for all living organisms. It can, therefore, be safely asserted that no plants, and therefore no living organisms, can live without the continuous activity of saprophytic micro-organisms. They effect chemical transformations of which neither plants nor animals are capable. Plants and animals cannot survive without the help of these micro-organisms. In their absence, all plants and animals would be destroyed.

The remaining two per cent of the micro-organisms are of the parasitic type. It is believed that they live on other living organisms. Their metabolic activities produce toxic substances in the bodies of other animals. This gives rise to various diseases. The famous scientist and bacteriologist, Louis Pasteur, was the originator of this belief. Exhilarated by this supposed discovery, Pasteur promptly declared that mankind could live thenceforward without fear of disease. But the sad fact is that he himself lived the rest of his life in constant fear of infection by bacteria. The spectre of this anxiety took possession of his mind to such an extent that he dared not eat even a banana without dipping it into boiling water, for fear that bacteria might possibly have burrowed through the skin

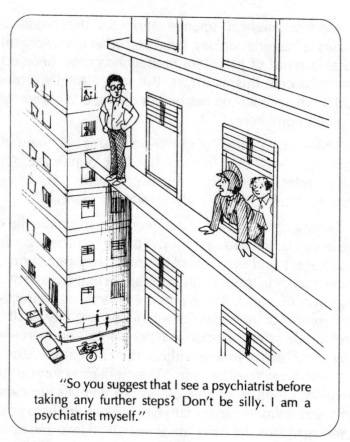

"So you suggest that I see a psychiatrist before taking any further steps? Don't be silly. I am a psychiatrist myself."

Fig. 5·1

of the banana! Once he inadvertently drank water that had been used to wash fresh grapes. When he realised the situation, he acted as if the sky had fallen. Unfortunately for the bacteria, he did not contract any disease on that occasion. But it is sad to reflect that Pasteur, who believed bacteria to be the sole cause of diseases, and who considered diet, exercise, etc. as of secondary importance, became the victim of hypertension, cerebral haemorrhage and paralysis in his middle age.

Is it true that most diseases are caused by infection due to bacteria? There are many doctors and bacteriologists that reject this view.

An eminent and learned Nature Cure practitioner Dr. Herbert Shelton confidently asserts that bacteria do not cause diseases, but on the contrary, it is only in diseased and toxic surroundings that they can carry on their noxious activities. It is only when our improper ways engender a poisonous environment, i.e., cause the accumulation of toxic materials, in our bodies that bacteria invade them to consume the poisons and thus remove them from the body. Eminent bacteriologists have supported this assertion. The famous British bacteriologist Sir Richard Douglas Powell discovered many years ago that the tetanus or gas gangrene germs lost their virulence when they were isolated from the diseased tissues. Thus the toxic nature of bacteria is dependent on toxic environment. It is only the accumulation of poisons in the body that provokes their virulence.

An important consideration is that if bacteria cause diseases, their presence in the body must precede the appearance of the symptoms of the disease. It is logical that cause should precede effect. But scientific investigations have made it clear time and again that bacteria have been found in bodies only after the symptoms have manifested themselves. **This indicates that the symptoms (and therefore the accumulation of toxic substances) are the cause, and the proliferation of bacteria the result,** and not the other way round.

Numerous investigations have shown that the supposedly dangerous bacteria do not cause diseases. Dr. Hunter's experiments in Australia point to the same conclusion. In one experiment, each of the subjects was given water containing 50 thousand germs of diphtheria. No effect was observed even after the lapse of several days. In the next experiment each subject was given 150 thousand of these germs in milk. Nothing happened to the subjects. In the third experiment a million germs of diphtheria were given to each subject in his food. There was no untoward effect. In the fourth experiment, millions of these germs were applied to the tonsils, the underside of the tongue and the mucous membranes of the nose. Even after this, no symptom of the disease could be observed. Similar experiments were tried with pneumonia and typhoid germs. In not a single instance could the germs produce the disease.

It is believed that the germs of the terrible disease meningitis proliferate especially in the mucous membranes of the nostrils. Special efforts were made in an experiment to test the effects of applying millions of meningitis germs to the mucous membranes of the nostrils, terbinate sinuses, tonsils, under the tongue and in the throat. No symptom of the disease was produced in a single case.

In the June, 1916 issue of the 'London Lancet Medical Journal of Canada', there is a report of an experiment performed by six doctors, in which germs of tuberculosis, diphtheria, pneumonia and typhoid were introduced by various means into the bodies of a number of subjects continuously for two and a half years, but no symptoms of any of the diseases were ever noticed.

The famous physician and professor of medicine at the Vienna University, Dr. Patinkoffer, came to the conclusion that germs just cannot cause diseases unaided. He publicised this belief through lectures and articles. He created a sensation among his students by drinking in their presence in the laboratory, a glass of water containing millions of cholera germs.

Dr. Thomas Powell of California, who lived to the ripe old age of eighty, voluntarily introduced more germs into his body than any other man. He had challenged his physician friends to make him ill by introducing any sort of germs in his body. Many bacteriologists took up the challenge and tried repeatedly, over a number of years, to prove him wrong. Germs of cholera, plague and other diseases were given to him in his food, injected into his veins, applied to his throat after scraping its mucous membrane; but Dr. Powell did not contract any of these diseases.

The attempts of Dr. Weit to murder Colonel Pack with the help of disease germs have become notorious. Dr. Weit kept on feeding the Colonel with supposedly lethal germs. But the intended victim appeared to flourish on this diet. At last Dr. Weit had to resort to chloroform and a cushion to dispose off the Colonel.

The gist of the above discussion is that Naturopathy does not attribute diseases to germs. It is impossible to keep germs away from our bodies. It has been found that 14,000 germs of tuberculosis, diphtheria, typhoid, cholera and other diseases enter the body of each one of us every hour through water, food and the air we breathe in. Why then do we not all contract all these diseases? It is obvious that if conditions in the body are not favourable for the growth and proliferation of these bacteria, they cannot cause diseases.

It requires only twenty minutes for one bacterium to grow and divide into two. In eight hours the number of descendants of one bacterium rises to 16 million, and in twenty-four hours to more than 5 billion (5 million million). This number of bacteria would be sufficient to destroy the whole human race. And this is just the progeny of a single bacterium. But we are ingesting 14,000 bacteria every hour! However, such phenomenal growth never actually occurs. If there is no food (poisons and wastes) for these bacteria in the body, they cannot flourish in the body, and eventually die out.

If, on the other hand, enough of such wastes and poisons are present in the body of any person, the bacteria begin to multiply. It must be remembered that so long as we do not refuse to provide bacteria with food and favourable conditions for growth, we are not likely to free ourselves from them. The residual bacteria in our bodies, and those that gain fresh entry into them, will keep on growing, as they find their food available in the body.

Attempts to destroy germs by the use of antibiotics are meaningless. To try to destroy the germs by poisoning them with antibiotics, instead of attacking the root cause of diseases, namely, the accumulated poisons in the body, would merely make the body a battleground for two different sets of toxic materials, which only results in harming the cells of the body and in weakening the Vital force. It makes no sense to risk grave side effects by consuming antibiotics to kill germs (which after all are not responsible for the disease) and incidentally to run the risk of grave side effects, even death. Hardly a hundred or a hundred and twenty-five years have passed, since doctors polished off hundreds of patients by administering large doses of the highly poisonous substance known as calomel. It was in the name of science that this terrible deed was done, and so was not looked upon as a crime. But today we condemr it in the strongest terms. More recently, penicillin has claimed not a few human lives, once again in the name of science. Many other medicines have been reported to cause equally serious side effects. Is it to be expected that the future generations will fail to condemn us for this irresponsible massacre in equally strong terms, and perhaps even worse?

According to Dr. Howard Winstein, the Director of the American Food and Drug Administration, some three to four thousand people become the victims of violent reactions to the administration of penicillin every year in the United States alone. Out of these, 300 to 400 incidents turn out to be fatal. The actual figures might well be much larger than these official ones. In many cases, the reactions and deaths caused by penicillin are blamed on the disease. Penicillin is used all over the world, in many countries without even testing for its reactions. One can form only a very rough estimate of the vast (staggering) world figures. There are many other drugs no less dangerous than penicillin, and numerous cases of reactions caused by them have been recorded. Despite all this, it continues to be argued by the proponents of drug therapy that after all, incidents of reactions are only few and far between. The truth of the matter is that all medicines have more or less adverse effects on the human body. They invariably weaken the Vital force.

An educated person may argue thus : (1) If germs do not cause diseases, how does an epidemic spread so quickly?

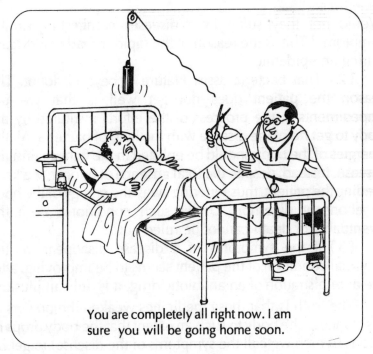

You are completely all right now. I am
sure you will be going home soon.

Fig. 5·2

(2) If germs really assist Nature in eliminating toxic
substances from the body, why do people die of diseases?
(3) Why is the condition of the patient found to improve after
the administration of antibiotics?

The contentions implied in these questions can be easily
refuted by a consideration of the facts, as shown in the
following answers to the questions, taken in order :

(1) It is axiomatic that identical causes produce
identical results. If we observe the individuals making up our
society with regard to their habits of eating and drinking,
breathing, sleeping, dressing, etc. and compare their
residences and their sporting activities and life-styles in
general, it will be obvious that in all respects there is a very
close resemblance. Now, if their life-styles are so similar,
would not all be equally weak and equally susceptible to
disease in the same manner? Would not the kinds and
amounts of poisons in their bodies also be closely similar?

Would not they suffer from diseases manifesting similar symptoms? This is the reason of the rapid spread of a disease during an epidemic.

(2) That bacteria assist Nature is beyond doubt. The reason the patient does not get well is that we put impediments in the progress of the efforts instituted by the body to get rid of the disease with the help of bacteria. All the energies of the body should be enlisted in the fight against the disease. Instead, despite the total absence of hunger, we keep feeding the patient, thus frittering away the energy of the body in efforts at digestion. Under such conditions, even the eventuality of death cannot be ruled out.

(3) If the symptoms of a disease disappear, or the physical condition of the patient seems to be improving, after the administration of an antibiotic drug, it is only an illusion.

The truth is that these medicines weaken the powers of resistance of the body to such an extent that the body drops its efforts (which we call the symptoms of the disease) to get rid of the disease. The acute disease, thus suppressed, turns chronic. In short, it is the attenuation of the symptoms under the action of the medicines that we construe as an improvement in the health of the patient.

Another basic principle of Nature Cure is that **it is Nature that heals, not the physician or the medicines.** In fact, the English word physician is derived from the Greek word 'Physis'. It means Nature. Unless and until the powers of resistance of the body are strengthened, it is not possible to cure the patient by the use of medicines, or indeed by any other method. That is precisely why all treatments in the Nature Cure system are directed to only one end : to strengthen the powers of resistance, i.e., the Vital force, of the body. Such treatments include diet, exercise, clay therapy, hydrotherapy, massage, sun-bathing, etc. These various types of treatment are discussed in the following chapters.

PART II : THE TOOLS OF NATUROPATHY

6. DIET

Is there a relation between diet and health? If so, what is the nature of this relation? There are few who can give convincing answers to these questions. The depth of our ignorance of these matters is really deplorable.

The attitude of allopathy towards diet is rather casual. It advises a 'balanced' diet, i.e., diet that contains the requisite proportions of proteins, carbohydrates, fats, vitamins and minerals. But most of the doctors are not much concerned about the diet of their patients. If a patient asks for advice in this regard, he is likely to be told that there are no specific restrictions : 'Eat everything......... within reason.'

Ayurveda has gone a little deeper into this question of the inter-relationship of diet and health. It classifies all foods into categories like phlegm-promoting or phlegm-destroying, bile-promoting or bile-destroying and gas-promoting or gas-destroying (that is, as related to the three humours of the body : कफ, पित्त, वात). To some extent, foods are also differentiated as 'heavy' or 'light' foods. Ayurveda had its origin thousands of years ago, when methods and equipment had not yet been developed for the analysis of foods. Ayurveda had no means of ascertaining what biochemical reactions took place in the body due to the ingestion of various foods. Its emphasis on the liberal consumption of ghee (clarified butter), oil, crystal sugar and spiced health-foods seems today to be a little outdated, and even misguided. There also seems to be an excessive bias in favour of cooked foods.

Diet is the mainstay of Naturopathic treatment. In this system, a detailed study has been made of the merits and demerits of each food and drink. Proper diet can be a veritable

43

elixir of life, lifting one to the pinnacle of health; improper diet, on the other hand, can act as a poison, destroying health and life. The views of Naturopathy concerning diet are discussed later on.

Food must serve two purposes : (1) Supply all essential nutrients to the body, and (2) maintain the acid-alkali balance in the blood.

Various foods, and how far they are suited to these purposes, are discussed in detail in the following paragraphs.

The body's requirements of essential nutrients : The five ingredients of foods essential for the nutrition of the body are : proteins, carbohydrates, fats, vitamins and minerals.

Proteins : Proteins are essential for the growth, maintenance and regeneration of the body. The main sources of proteins are pulses, milk, eggs, meat, etc. All proteins are made up of amino acids and different proteins contain different proportions of the various amino acids.

There are in all twenty-three amino acids in food proteins. Out of these, there are ten that the human body cannot synthesize : arginine, histidine, isoleucine, leucine, lysine, methionine, phenylalanine, threonine, tryptophane and valine. These are, therefore, called 'essential' amino acids. The body must be supplied with the requisite amounts of these amino acids through food. The rest of the amino acids can be synthesized by the body from these. The functions of each of the amino acids in the body are set out in the following table, along with their vegetable sources.

No.	Amino Acid	The Part of the Body for Which it is Needed	Sources
1	Alanine	Skin, adrenal glands	Alfalfa, carrots, celery, lettuce, cucumber, turnips, green pepper, spinach, apples, plums, guavas, grapes, oranges, strawberries, almonds.

No.	Amino Acid	The Part of the Body for Which it is Needed	Sources
2	Arginine	Muscles, cartilage cells, reproductive organs, prevention of senility	Alfalfa, green leafy vegetables, carrots, beetroots, cucumber, celery, lettuce, radishes, potatoes.
3	Aspartic acid	Bones, teeth, lungs, heart, blood vessels	Carrots, celery, cucumber, mint, radishes, tomatoes, turnips, lemons, grapefruit, apples, plums, pineapples, melons, almonds.
4	Cystine	Hair, erythrocytes, breasts, vitality	Alfalfa, carrots, beetroots, cabbages, cauliflower, onions, garlic, apples, pineapples, raspberries, raisins.
5	Glutamic acid	Pancreas, secretion of digestive juices, prevention of anaemia	Carrots, turnips, cabbages, celery, beetroots, mint, lettuce, spinach, papaya.
6	Glycine	Cartilage cells, muscles, secretion of sex hormones	Carrots, turnips, celery, mint, spinach, alfalfa, garlic, potatoes, figs, oranges, raspberries, pomegranates, melons, almonds.
7	Histidine	Liver, haemoglobin, semen	Radishes, carrots, beetroots, celery, cucumber, garlic, onions, turnips, alfalfa, spinach, apples, pineapples, pomegranates, papaya.
8	Hydroxy-glutamic acid	Secretion of digestive juices	Carrots, mint, lettuce, spinach, tomatoes, grapes, raspberries, plums.
9	Hydroxy proline	Liver, gall bladder, erythrocytes	Carrots, beetroots, lettuce, turnips, cucumber, plums, cherries, figs, radishes, grapes, olives, pineapples, almonds, coconuts.
10	Iodogorgoic acid	Various glands	Carrots, celery, spinach, tomatoes, lettuce, pineapples.

No.	Amino Acid	The Part of the Body for Which it is Needed	Sources
11	Isoleucine	Thymus, spleen, pituitary gland, haemoglobin, regulation of metabolism	Papaya, olives, coconuts, almonds, apricots, pistachios, walnuts.
12	Leucine	Counterbalancing isoleucine	As in No. 11.
13	Lysine	Liver, gall bladder, fat metabolism, various processes in the body, prevention of senility	Carrots, beetroots, cucumber, celery, mint, spinach, turnips, alfalfa, germinated soyabeans, papaya, apples, plums, pears, grapes.
14	Methionine	Haemoglobin, spleen, pancreas	Cabbages, cauliflower, garlic, pineapples, apples.
15	Norleucine	Counterbalancing leucine	—
16	Phenylalanine	Elimination of foreign substances, kidneys, urinary bladder	Carrots, beetroots, spinach, mint, tomatoes, pineapples, apples.
17	Proline	White blood corpuscles (leucocytes)	Carrots, beetroots, lettuce, turnips, cucumber, plums, cherries, figs, grapes, olives, oranges, pineapples, coconuts, almonds.
18	Serine	Mucous membranes, lungs, bronchi	Radishes, garlic, onions, carrots, beetroots, celery, cucumber, mint, spinach, cabbage, alfalfa, papaya, apples, pineapples.
19	Threonine	To make good the deficiency of some other amino acids	Carrots, alfalfa, green leafy vegetables, papaya.
20	Thyroxine	Thyroid, pituitary glands, adrenal glands, regulation of metabolism	Carrots, celery, lettuce, spinach, turnips, tomatoes, pineapples.
21	Tryptophane	Regeneration of cells, secretion of digestive juices, eyes	Carrots, beetroots, celery, spinach, alfalfa, turnips.

No.	Amino Acid	The Part of the Body for Which it is Needed	Sources
22	Tyrosine	Erythrocytes, leuco-cytes, hair; adrenal, pituitary and thyroid glands	Alfalfa, carrots, beetroots, cucumber, lettuce, mint, spinach, green pepper, plums, strawberries, cherries, apples, melons, figs, almonds.
23	Valine	Breasts, ovaries	Carrots, turnips, sweet gourd, celery, mint, beetroots, tomatoes, apples, pomegranates, almonds.

Many nutritionists believe that animal proteins are superior and indeed complete food proteins, or 'first class' proteins, whereas vegetable proteins are inferior, incomplete and 'second class' proteins. This belief is based on the fact that meat contains all the essential amino acids, but any one specific vegetable food does not contain all of them. They, therefore, advise people to take meat in one form or the other. They insist on vegetarians taking plenty of milk, so that they can get sufficient amounts of superior proteins and the body can be maintained at its best.

But this insistence on animal proteins, whether in the form of meat or milk, is misguided. By combining vegetable proteins in proper proportions, we can get all the essential amino acids in the requisite amounts. One food may lack lysine, but may contain enough of tryptophane. Another one may lack tryptophane, but may supply all the lysine required. Thus by a judicious blending of foodstuffs, the deficiency of any amino acid can be compensated for. For instance, if wheaten foods are combined with vegetables, the combination yields 'first class' proteins – proteins of the best quality. In fine, there is no justification for the belief that a vegetarian is likely to suffer from the deficiency of one or more essential amino acids. That superior proteins are available in animal food is beyond question, but it must be remembered that there are numerous drawbacks attached to the use of such foods.

A non-vegetarian diet provides excessive amounts of proteins to the body. And excess of proteins is unquestionably the chief factor in the causation of many diseases. The famous dietician, Dr. Chittenden, states that **"ingestion of excessive amounts of proteins results in the formation of uric acid, which is harmful to health. Many of the diseases troubling mankind have their roots in the excessive intake of proteins."**

In the opinion of Dr. Hindheed, when too much of protein enters the blood stream, it gets converted into nitric acid, sulphuric acid and phosphoric acid. The body is forced to use up large amounts of alkali minerals to neutralize these acids. This results in a deficiency of minerals in the bones, hair and nails. The acids mentioned above cause so much damage to the liver and the kidneys that in some cases it may even prove fatal.

Dr. Hindheed has studied the food habits of various communities. He concluded that diseases are less prevalent in countries where the consumption of proteinous foods is low. He got an opportunity to amass evidence in support of this conclusion during the First World War.

At that time he was Food Administrator in Denmark. He could reduce the death-rate among the Danes by 40 per cent through a drastic reduction in the per capita consumption of proteins. Dr. Hindheed forcefully asserted that no adult wishing to live a long and healthy life should take more than twenty grammes of proteins per day. This admonition sounds a warning note against the exhortations of some dieticians to take 60 to 100 grammes of proteins daily.

Dr. J. H. Kellogg, the founder of the famous Battle-Creek Sanatorium, attributes the rise in the proportion of deaths due to Bright's disease in America and other developed countries solely to excessive consumption of meat, which is, of course, rich in proteins.

Dr. Squire and Dr. Newberg thoroughly investigated the effect of protein-rich foods on the kidneys. In one experiment they began to feed each of five healthy men half a kilogramme of meat every day. Before the commencement of the experiment there was nothing unusual in the urine of these men. But within a few days of the start of the experiment, erythrocytes and albumin were detected in the urine of each.

In this connection it is worth noting that Dr. Chittenden found that reducing the proportion of proteins in the diet results in an increase in the physical and mental energy, a capacity to work for long periods without getting tired, and reduced susceptibility to disease.

There is another point that deserves consideration. Meat contains a relatively larger proportion of the amino acid methionine. Many investigators believe that, if methionine is not metabolised properly in the body, the ultimate results are the development of atherosclerosis and the consequent increased risk of heart attack. Meat also contains large amounts of cholesterol. And vegetarians (lactovegetarians) should keep it in mind that as milk is an animal product, it is not free from the above drawbacks.

Carbohydrates : Carbohydrates provide heat and energy to the body. Cereals, tubers, roots, pulses, milk, etc. are the main sources of carbohydrates.

There can be no objection to the use of natural carbo-hydrates in their original forms. But the use of processed carbohydrates is not desirable. De-branned flour, polished rice, white flour, refined sugar, etc. are instances of such processed foods. Processing removes the fibres and roughage from the food. This results in insufficient elimination of wastes. Toxic substances consequently accumulate in the blood. We cause a lot of damage to our health by consuming canned and bottled fruits, fruit juices, tomato ketchup, jams, jellies, instant gulabjamuns, instant rasagullas, ready-ground flours, cakes, chocolates, icecream, bread, biscuits, peppermint sweets and other similar processed carbohydrates. As such foods are easily overeaten, the digestive organs are subjected to undesirably heavy loads. The consequence is severe indigestion and obesity, resulting later in more or less permanent diseased conditions like diabetes, or disorders of the joints.

Fats : Fats, too, like carbohydrates, perform the function of supplying heat and energy to the body. Ghee (clarified butter) and oils are the main sources of fats for vegetarians.

There are two types of fats : Saturated and unsaturated. Prolonged use of saturated fats causes constriction and hardening of the arteries, which may result in hypertension, heart-attack and other related ailments. It is, therefore, necessary to minimise the intake of saturated fats, replacing them, if at all necessary, by unsaturated fats.

Lists of foods containing saturated and unsaturated fats are given in the following table :

Foods containing saturated fats	Foods containing unsaturated fats
(a) Butter, ghee (clarified butter), vegetable ghee, coconut oil, palm oil.	Peanut oil, seasame oil, maize oil, soyabean oil, karadi oil, cottonseed oil, sunflower oil, and dishes prepared from these oils.
(b) Whole-milk, cream, khoya, khoya-based preparations, sweets prepared in ghee and vegetable ghee, whole-milk preparations (shreekhand, basudi, ice-cream, pedas, etc.).	
(c) Chocolates, cakes, biscuits, wafers.	
(d) Eggs, fat meat, oysters, fish.	

The following table shows the amounts of fats and cholesterol in various foodstuffs :

Amounts of Fats and Cholesterol in Foods

Food	Approximate Quantity	Weight Grammes	Total Fats Grammes	Saturated Fats Grammes	Unsaturated Fats		Cholesterol milligrammes
					Oleic Acid Grammes	Linoleic Acid Grammes	
1. Liver	1 Oz	30	1·5	0·4	Trace	Trace	75
2. Bacon	1½ Oz	40	17·6	6·4	7·6	1·6	45
3. Egg	1	50	6·0	2·0	2·5	0·5	253
4. Oyster	1 Oz	30	1·9	0·6	1·0	0·3	45
5. Whole-Milk	1 Cup	240	8·5	4·9	3·6	–	27
6. Skimmed-Milk	1 Cup	240	–	–	–	–	7
7. Cake	1 Piece	50	14·0	2·0	–	0·5	45
8. Biscuit	1	35	6·5	2·3	3·4	0·8	17
9. Icecream	½ Cup	75	9·0	5·0	3·9	–	43
10. Butter	1 Teaspoon	5	4·0	2·3	1·2	–	12
11. Coconut Oil	1 Teaspoon	5	5·0	4·4	0·5	0·1	–
12. Karadi Oil	1 Teaspoon	5	5·0	0·4	1·0	3·6	–
13. Cottonseed Oil	1 Teaspoon	5	5·0	1·3	1·2	2·5	–
14. Peanut Oil	1 Teaspoon	5	5·0	0·9	1·6	2·5	–
15. Maize Oil	1 Teaspoon	5	5·0	0·5	1·8	2·7	–
16. Soyabean Oil	1 Teaspoon	5	5·0	0·8	1·6	2·6	–
17. Seasame Oil	1 Teaspoon	5	5·0	0·9	1·0	2·1	–

Vitamins and Minerals : The body needs only minute quantities of these substances, but they are of great importance. They perform various important functions in the body. Vitamins are essential for the proper digestion and absorption of proteins, carbohydrates and fats, and the development of the ability of the body to protect itself against diseases. Various minerals are needed for the formation and functioning of the cells. These vital substances are necessary for the maintenance of health. They are all the more necessary in sickness. Various disorders are the direct results of the deficiency of vitamins and minerals.

The stores of the vitamins in the body get quickly depleted during an illness. Improper diet, mental distress, pollution, smoking, addiction to drugs are other factors that destroy the vitamins in the body. In an investigation it has been established that smoking one cigarette destroys about 25 milligrammes of vitamin C. Other vitamins are also destroyed in analogous ways. On the other hand, the requirements of vitamins have increased manifold these days due to the mental stresses and worries which have become so common in modern times. Unwholesome diet and the uninhibited use of medicines such as sulpha drugs, antibiotics and cortisones also tend to reduce the reserves of vitamins in the body.

It is clear from the above considerations that man needs vitamins and minerals today as never before. Adequate quantities of these essential components of foods are available in uncooked foods, germinated grains and beans, as well as in fruits, vegetables and their juices.

Cooking destroys vitamins. The vitamins in fruits and vegetables are rapidly lost if they are not consumed immediately after peeling or cutting them.

Some dieticians contend that Vitamin B_{12} can be obtained only from meat. But they forget that meat is not eaten raw, and cooking destroys most of the Vitamin B_{12} in it.

The vitamins in natural foodstuffs are in a 'live' and easily digestible form, and so are quickly and completely assimilated in the body. On the other hand, experiments have decisively proved that the expected benefit is almost never afforded by the use of synthetic vitamins in the forms of tablets, pills, etc. In the same way, the body cannot satisfactorily utilise artificially synthesised or purified mineral salts. In short, if the body lacks minerals, the deficiency cannot be made good by medicines.

Functions of Vitamins and Minerals : The functions of vitamins and minerals and their sources, as also the ailments caused by their deficiencies are set out in the following tables:

VITAMINS

Vitamin	Daily Requirement of an Adult	Function	Sources	Symptoms of Deficiency
Vitamin A	4000 to 5000 International Units (I.U.)	This vitamin is necessary for the development and protection of certain cells in the body. It is essential for a healthy condition of the eyes. Night vision is also dependent on it. It is needed for the development of bones and formation of teeth as well.	Milk, cheese, butter, green leafy vegetables, cabbages, carrots, red and yellow fruits and vegetables. Large amounts of Vitamin A are also found in fish liver oils (e.g. cod liver oil).	Vitamin A deficiency slows down growth, causes dryness of skin and eyes, eventually leading to night blindness; deformation of bones and teeth may also result.
Vitamin B Note: This is actually a group of vitamins comprising eight vitamins: Vitamin B_1, Vitamin B_2, Niacin, Vitamin B_6, Pantothenic Acid, Biotin, Folcin and Vitamin B_{12}	0·5 to 5 mg of each vitamin of this group	This group of vitamins is necessary for the development of the body, appetite, healthy condition of eyes, nerves and skin, and for the prevention of anaemia.	Milk, yeast, wheat bran, germinated wheat, leafy vegetables, fresh vegetables and fruits, pulses, etc. are the usual sources. It is also present in eggs, meat (especially liver), and fish.	Vitamin B_1 deficiency causes beri-beri. Deficiency of Vitamin B_2 causes chaps on the skin around the eyes, nose and mouth. Niacin deficiency is responsible for pellagra and deterioration of nerves. Insufficient intake of Vitamin B_6 results in anaemia and skin diseases. Metabolic reactions are disrupted by a lack of pantothenic acid. The symptoms of deficiency of biotin or folcin resemble those caused by a lack of pantothenic acid. Deficiency of Vitamin B_{12} slows down growth and induces pernicious anaemia.

VITAMINS

Vitamin	Daily Requirement of an Adult	Function	Sources	Symptoms of Deficiency
Vitamin C	45 mg	This vitamin is essential for the proper development of the body. It also helps the formation of bones and teeth. It helps various cells to cohere together, heals wounds, augments the resistance of the body to diseases, and is also a factor in the synthesis of steroid hormones in the body.	Sources of Vitamin C include sweet-sour fruits, myrobalan, tomatoes, watermelons, pears, cabbages, pineapples, potatoes and green leafy vegetables.	Lack of Vitamin C causes scurvy, diseased conditions of teeth and gums, internal haemorrhage, osteoporosis, loss of weight, and in some cases, even sterility.
Vitamin D	300 to 400 I.U.	This vitamin is necessary for the development of the body. It plays an important part in the formation of bones and teeth.	Sunlight is the best source of Vitamin D. It also occurs in milk, eggs and some fish liver oils.	Osteoporesis is caused by deficiency of Vitamin D. This leads to rickets in children.
Vitamin E	12 to 15 I.U.	This vitamin is important for the reproductive function. In addition, it strengthens the erythrocytes and prevents their fragmentation.	Milk, germinated wheat, green leafy vegetables, vegetable oils, nuts and eggs are sources of this vitamin.	Lack of this vitamin may cause sterility.
Vitamin K	1 to 2 mg	It is essential for the production of prothrombin, which is responsible for the clotting of blood.	It is found in wheat bran, green leafy vegetables, tomatoes, cauliflower, soyabean oil, vegetable oils, and livers of animals.	If there is a deficiency of this vitamin, prothrombin cannot be synthesized by the body. As a result, blood fails to clot, and even minor cuts result in copious bleeding.

MINERALS

Mineral	Daily Requirement of an Adult	Function	Sources	Probable Symptoms of Deficiency
Calcium	800 mg	99% of calcium in the body is found in bones and teeth. It is also necessary for the transport of some substances into or out of cells.	Milk and milk products, *methi*, drumsticks, and other green leafy vegetables, beetroots, figs, grapes, watermelons, millets, seasame and black grams are good sources of calcium. Some fish and oysters also contain plenty of calcium.	Lack of calcium weakens bones and teeth, and causes osteoporesis.
Phosphorus	800 mg	About 80% of the phosphorus in the body is present in the bones and teeth. It is an important constituent of every cell. It helps to regulate the pH of the blood, and is necessary for the formation of substances like DNA, RNA, ATP, which are essential for life processes.	Milk, cheese, yeast, dry fruits, soyabeans, dates, carrots, guava, etc. are the sources of phosphorus. It is also present in eggs, fish and meat.	Lack of phosphorus causes weakening of the bones and teeth, and loss of weight.
Potassium	2500 mg	Potassium is an important constituent of cellular fluid. It is required for the metabolism of carbohydrates and proteins. It helps in the regulation of the pH of the blood.	Plenty of potassium is supplied by fresh fruits, milk, garlic, radishes, potatoes and meat.	Potassium deficiency may cause weakness of the muscles, even paralysis. It may also cause brittleness of the bones, sterility and heart ailments.

MINERALS

Mineral	Daily Require- ment of an Adult	Function	Sources	Probable Symptoms of Deficiency
Sodium	2500 mg	Sodium is an important constituent of the extra-cellular fluids. 30 to 40% sodium is present in the bones.	Common salt, milk, beetroots, carrots, radishes, *phanasi* etc. contain sodium. It is also present in eggs, meat and fish.	Lack of sodium can cause headache, nausea, slower development of the body, and disorders of the muscles.
Iron	10 mg	Nearly 70% of the iron in the body is present in haemoglobin in red blood cells. 26% iron is stored in the liver, spleen and bones. In the absence of iron, the cells cannot take up oxygen or eliminate carbon dioxide.	*Methi*, mint and other green leafy vegetables, seasame, millets, grams, green grams, black grams, soyabeans, dates, mangoes, etc. are good sources of iron. So are eggs, meat, animal livers, oysters, etc.	Anaemia is the principal symptom of iron deficiency.
Sulphur	300 mg	Sulphur is a constituent of proteins, and some vitamins. It is also required for metabolic processes.	Beetroots, cabbage, radishes, garlic, onions, milk and meat are the sources of sulphur.	Some metabolic processes in the body are hindered by a deficiency of sulphur.
Magnesium	350 mg	Nearly 50% magnesium is found in the bones and the remaining 50% in the cells. Magnesium is necessary for the activation of many enzymes. Hence a large number of processes taking place in the body are dependent on magnesium.	Milk, cereals, green vegetables, dry fruit and meat contain magnesium.	Bones, teeth and muscles weaken due to the deficiency of magnesium. Insufficient supply of magnesium may even give rise to heart ailments.

MINERALS

Mineral	Daily Requirement of an Adult	Function	Sources	Probable Symptoms of Deficiency
Chlorine	2000 mg	This element functions in association with sodium. It is one of the main constituents of extra-cellular fluids. It activates certain enzymes. It is a constituent of the digestive juices of the stomach.	Common salt, milk, carrots, *phanasi*, potatoes, spinach, cabbage, tomatoes, bananas, dates, etc. contain chlorine. Chlorine is also present in eggs, meat and salt-water fish also.	Bones weaken and joints stiffen if there is a deficiency of chlorine.
Iodine	0·14 mg	It is a constituent of the secretion of the thyroid gland.	It is present in sea foods and green vegetables.	Lack of iodine impairs the function of the thyroid gland, resulting in goitre.

Acid and Alkali Balance in Blood : The ratio of acids to alkalis in blood is generally 20 : 80. Maintenance of this ratio is essential for health. The body naturally exerts its utmost to maintain this ratio.

Some of our foods leave alkaline residues in the body after undergoing the full cycle of digestive and metabolic processes; some others leave acidic residues. We may call such foods alkali-genic and acid-genic respectively. Generally, the acids produced by the metabolic activities, (such as uric acid, lactic acid, etc.) react with the alkalis in the blood, lymph, bile, etc., thus being neutralised and rendered innocuous. But if our diet is replete with acid-genic foods, the body cannot cope with all the resulting acids. When the acids accumulate in the blood, symptoms associated with acidic blood like fatigue, headache, anorexia, insomnia, nervous tension, hyperacidity, coryza, etc., begin to appear.

Acidic blood is an abnormal condition that hinders the physical development of children and adolescents, causes degeneration in older people, and diminishes vitality. It causes difficulties in pregnancy and lactation. It is the origin of diseases like measles, appendicitis, pneumonia, tuberculosis and cancer.

Dr. George Cryle, the renowned surgeon of Cleveland, USA, is of the firm opinion that there is no such thing as natural death. All so-called natural deaths are the culminating stages of chronic acidic condition of the blood.

The above discussion makes it quite clear that all the toxic substances in the body are in the form of acids, and that in order to prevent or counteract the accumulation of acids in the body we must take food that is mainly alkali-genic.

It is important, therefore, know what food will result in the generation of how much alkalinity or acidity in the body. The well-known Biochemist Dr. Regnar Burg has carried out extensive investigations regarding the overall acidic or alkaline effects of various foods.

A table based on his results is presented here :

ALKALI-GENIC FOODS		ACID-GENIC FOODS	
Food	Alkali-genic effect in per cent	Food	Acid-genic effect in per cent
FRUITS :		**CEREALS :**	
Figs (fresh)	27·81	Rice (polished)	17·96
Raisins	15·10	Rice (manually de-husked)	3·68
Grapes	7·15		
Sugar-cane	14·57	Cake	12·31
Tomatoes	13·67	Bread	10·99
Lemons	9·90	Barley	10·58
Oranges	9·61	White Flour (Wheat)	8·32
Plums	5·80	Maize	5·37
Dates	5·50	Wheat	2·66
Peaches	5·40	**PULSES AND LEGUMES :**	
Apricots (fresh)	4·79		
Bananas	4·38	All pulses and legumes	
Pomegranates	4·15	Highly acid-genic	
Coconuts	4·09	**NUTS :**	
Pineapples	3·59		
Pears	3·26	Peanuts	16·39
Watermelons	1·83	Walnuts	9·22
Apples	1·38	Almonds	2·19
VEGETABLES, TUBERS AND ROOTS :		**FOOD OF ANIMAL ORIGIN (EXCLUDING MILK) :**	
Spinach	28·01		
Suva Plants	18·36	Yolk of Egg	51·83
Leafy Salad Plants	14·12	White of Egg	8·27
Cucumbers	13·50	Eggs	11·61
Beetroots	11·37	Beef	38·61
Turnips	10·80	Chicken	24·32
Sweet Potatoes (Yams)	10·31	Goat's Flesh	20·30
Radishes	6·05	Fish	19·52
Potatoes	5·90	Pork	12·47
Peas (fresh)	5·15	**MILK PRODUCTS :**	
Cabbage	4·02		
Cauliflower	3·04	Cheese	17·49
Onions	1·09	Butter	4·33
Pumpkin	0·28		
MILK AND MILK PRODUCTS :			
Skimmed Milk	4·89		
Cream	2·66		
Human Milk	2·25		
Cow's Milk	1·69		
Butter Milk	1·31		
Goat's Milk	0·25		

From the table it is obvious that meat, fish, eggs and pulses are highly acid-genic. Wholemeal wheat flour, manually dehusked unpolished rice, and such other cereals in their more or less natural forms are only mildly acid-genic, but processing or refining them makes them much more acidic in effect. All vegetables, tubers, roots and fruits are alkali-genic. Green leafy vegetables are of special importance in this respect.

Let us think of our traditional daily fare in the context of this table. For breakfast we usually take milk, tea, coffee, khakhras, buns, chiwda, ganthias, biscuits, etc. All these foods are acid-genic. Dal, rice and chapaties, which are the mainstays of the mid-day meal, are also highly acid-genic. Only the vegetables are alkali-genic. But even in their case the alkalis have been rendered ineffective by oxidation during the process of cooking. Refreshments in the afternoon also consist of tea and fried preparations, or in some cases sandwiches, idlis, dosas, etc. Most of these are again acid-forming. Rice, dal, curry, khichdi, bhakhris, which comprise the usual evening meal are all acid-genic foods. The enormous amounts of the alkalis stored in the body which are wasted in counteracting this onslaught of acids can only be conjectured. We have not formed habits of regularly taking alkali-genic foods like fruits. And we have not realized the importance of uncooked vegetables at all. It is chiefly for this reason that our entire nation is caught up in the web of diseases and medicines.

It is quite possible to maintain a balance between the acids and alkalis in the body by a judicious combination of various unprocessed cereals, raw vegetables, fruits and nuts in our daily diet and thus keep diseases at bay. Not only do the alkalis in such foods neutralize the acids in other foods, but they also help in extracting the acids and toxins accumulated in the cells of the body, and ejecting them from the system. These qualities make a diet made up of alkali-genic components not only pure and wholesome, but also an efficient eliminating and cleansing agency.

Life, it is universally acknowledged, begets life; it would not be reasonable, therefore, to expect that food consisting of dead matter can enliven the body. But cooking our food, and thus rendering it lifeless, has become an established convention. We keep doing what our forebears used to do. No other animal subsists on cooked food, and though domesticated animals like dogs, cats and cows may find cooked food acceptable, still if given a free choice they would always instinctively prefer raw uncooked food.

The human body is subjected to constant wear and tear. Cells die, and are replaced by new ones. These processes of regeneration require vitamins, mineral salts and enzymes. Vitamins and enzymes are also necessary for the digestion and assimilation of proteins, carbohydrates, fats, etc. These enzymes and some of the vitamins are destroyed by heat. As a consequence they are not available in adequate amounts in cooked foods.

Food is a necessity for the body, not for the tongue. Meals planned with only the titillation of the taste buds as the principal aim are scarcely suitable for the nutrition of the body. Spices may vastly improve the taste of foods, so that we consume them with alacrity and enthusiasm, but that is hardly the only or the main purpose of taking food. We eat to live, and do not—or should not—live to eat. And we need not disregard taste completely : proper combinations of the natural flavours can make even uncooked foods tasty and appetising.

Cooking not only destroys vitamins and enzymes in the foods, but also results in degradation of their nutritive value. Proteins in foods are coagulated and hardened by cooking. Such coagulated proteins are not digested, but decay in the digestive tract. Cooking also makes carbohydrates less easy to digest. As a result, they are not absorbed completely in the intestines. Thus in terms of nutrients our cooked foods are comparatively almost valueless. A healthy person may still be able to extract the residual nutrients from them, but this is hardly possible for one who is ailing, and whose need for them is, therefore, greater.

The notion that raw food is indigestible, and will cause heaviness in the belly, stomach ache or gas, is erroneous. It has been established by experiments that cooked foods require five to six hours for complete digestion, while raw foods need only three to four hours. Fruit and vegetable juices are digested, and begin to get absorbed, in only twenty-five to thirty minutes. Thus uncooked food, and especially uncooked liquid food, affords rest for the digestive organs. The valuable energy of the body is not wasted in useless, futile attempts at digesting the indigestible, and thus becomes available for regeneration and healing.

Cooking, as we have seen, destroys valuable constituents of foods. But, on the other hand, germination of grain and pulses results in a vast increase in their nutritive contents. In uncooked germinated seeds, there is an increase of up to 600 per cent in the amounts of thiamin (Vitamin B_1), pantothenic acid, niacin, etc., and that too in a natural, live form. The number of yeast cells, so useful to the body, increases by 6 thousand million. Lactation in nursing mothers increases considerably by the consumption of germinated cereals and pulses. This naturally leads to the proper and quicker development of the child as well.

An experiment of Dr. Alexis Carrel, the author of 'Man, the Unknown' and the President of the Rockefeller Institute, is very significant in this context. Dr. Carrel kept some cells from the heart of a hen alive for thirty years in vegetable juice. When the experiment was terminated at the end of the thirtieth year, the cells were still perfectly healthy and active. Dr. Carrel claimed that the experiment could have been continued for 100 or even 1000 years, because the cells showed absolutely no signs of ageing or degeneration. If cells can be kept alive for such a long period outside the body, it should be much easier to do so within the body. It is no exaggeration then to say that by proper nutrition it should be possible to keep the human body, too, alive and active for correspondingly long periods.

Dr. George J. Druce of Chicago, USA, has remarked very significantly that cooked food is the oldest addiction of mankind. 95 per cent of physical and mental disorders are the products of such lifeless food.

Food Combinations for Easy Digestion : Only if we understand and act in accordance with the rules of food combinations can we hope for proper digestion. If these rules are violated, even good nutritious food may produce toxic materials as a result of decomposition in the digestive tract. For instance, there is no enzyme in the stomach which can digest carbohydrates. Carbohydrates are digested either in the mouth or in the small intestine. On the other hand, the digestion of proteins takes place in the stomach. Let us consider a meal that contains large quantities of both carbohydrates and proteins. If it is masticated properly, the enzymes in the saliva in the mouth carry out partial digestion of the carbohydrates. But if the food is swallowed without adequate mastication, the carbohydrates will remain undigested in the stomach while the proteins are being digested. They will, therefore, decay and produce toxic materials. Consider chapaties, for instance. If a morsel of chapaty is chewed well, the carbohydrates in it will be converted into sugars, imparting a sweet taste to the morsel. These sugars are absorbed directly into the blood stream as soon as they reach the stomach. Now if the chapaties are not chewed properly, the carbohydrates are in a completely undigested condition, with the result that they start decaying in the stomach. An important point to be noted is that the enzymes in the saliva can act only in an alkaline medium. If sour chutneys or pickles are taken along with a morsel of the chapaty, or if the vegetable or dal taken with the chapaty contain limes, tomatoes, tamarind or similar sources of acids, the enzymes in the saliva get de-activated, and therefore completely undigested carbohydrates find their way into the stomach. It is, therefore, advisable not to take chapaties and sour foods simultaneously. Mixing them can only lead to the production of toxic substances in the body.

Rules for the selection of food combinations are given' below :

(1) Carbohydrates should never be mixed with sour foods. This has been explained at length in the preceding paragraphs.

(2) Large amounts of proteins and large amounts of carbohydrates should not be taken in the same meal. The reasons for this rule too have been explained earlier.

(3) Large amounts of proteins should not be taken simultaneously with large amounts of fats (e.g. dal and ghee). The reason is the same as for the above rules : these two types of foods are digested in different parts of the digestive tract.

(4) Proteinous foods should not be ingested with sour fruits. For instance, if lemon juice or tomatoes are added to dal, the acids in these fruits cause a diminution in the secretion of digestive juices, rendering digestion less efficient.

These rules apply with greater force to people with weaker constitution or weaker digestive powers. People in robust health may not suffer any serious ill effects by ingesting foods in improper combinations. It is also a fact that Nature itself has combined carbohydrates and proteins, or proteins and fats, together in many foods; it is not possible to effect a separation of these constituents.

In the diagram captioned 'Food Combinations' various classes of foods are shown along with indications as to which combinations of these foods are beneficial, and which are harmful.

Ideal Daily Schedule of Alimentation :

(1) **Early morning :** Lemon juice (of one lemon or half a lemon) in a glass of water. People suffering from a cold should take the juice in warm water. No sugar, salt or honey must be added.

(2) **8·30 to 9·30 in the morning :** Fruits or fruit juice; bananas, dates, raisins, dry fruit and similar nutritious foods may also be taken.

FOOD COMBINATIONS

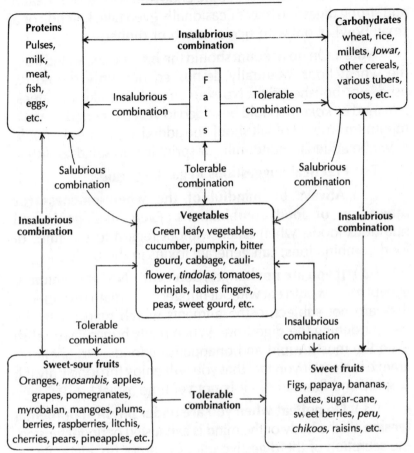

(3) **Lunch :** Begin with half a cup of the uncooked juice of leafy vegetables, or a cup of soup of such vegetables. This can be followed by some germinated pulses, some raw vegetables, and if desired, some sweet-sour fruits—all to be masticated well. The meal may be concluded with wheat chapaties and boiled vegetables. Rice can be substituted for the chapaties. Occasionally, the meal may be topped off with buttermilk. In indifferent health, avoid the pulses.

(4) **3·00 to 4·00 in the afternoon :** Fruits, or fruit juice.

(5) **Dinner :** As for lunch, except that the uncooked juice of vegetables should be omitted. The chapaties may be made from other cereals. People endowed with robust health and strong digestion may occasionally even take khichdi; or a small bowl of dal with rice at lunch or dinner.

Note : On no account should the bran be separated from the wheat flour. Manually de-husked rice only should be used, not polished rice. No sour ingredients like tomatoes, tamarind or *kokum* should be added to vegetables or dal, and a minimum amount of salt should be added to them. Salt should never be added to buttermilk, or sprinkled on salads or fruits.

Ten Practical Suggestions Regarding Food :

(1) **Always be mindful of the wholesomeness (or otherwise) of food combinations :** Even alkali-genic and nutritious foods, when taken without regard to the rules of food combinations, can generate toxins in the body.

(2) **If you are not hungry, don't eat :** No other animals, except man, would eat without hunger—the main reason why they are not subject to the ailments which man invites by overburdening the digestion. When really hungry, we relish even the most insipid and unappetising foods. Dr. Shelton's advice is clear: If you feel that you will enjoy the food only if it is spicy and flavoured,— it is not yet time to eat!

(3) **Do not eat when you are under physical or mental tension :** If the body or the mind is exhausted or under tension, the secretion of the digestive juices will not be adequate.

(4) **Do not eat or drink anything that is too hot or too cold :** Ideally the temperature of any food should be around 37°C (98.6° F), the temperature of the body. The enzymes in the mouth and the stomach act best at such temperatures.

(5) **Chew your food well :** Thorough chewing mixes saliva with the food. Digestion starts off in the mouth itself with the action of the enzymes present in the saliva. Moreover, well-chewed food is easily digested.

(6) **Do not drink water with meals :** Water requires only ten minutes to be absorbed from the stomach, and in the process it carries the enzymes away. This reduces the efficiency of the digestive process, which may result in the loss of appetite. There is no objection to drinking water fifteen minutes before a meal, half an hour after taking fruits, and two hours after a full meal.

(7) **Do not stuff the belly with food** : Overeating is always harmful. The stomach is a flexible bag made up of muscles. Its rhythmic contractions and expansions are responsible for the efficient mixing of digestive juices and enzymes with food. These movements are hindered if the bag is stuffed up with excessive food. The enzymes are not mixed properly with the food, which begins to decay. Most people fail to exercise discretion in the amount of food they take. They seem to live for eating, and not to eat for living ! Overeating makes one lethargic and dull. There is a constant feeling of thirst. With time the belly gets enlarged, and one falls victim to disorders of the digestive system. In fact, to keep healthy it is necessary at all times to remain slightly hungry.

(8) **Rest for a while after meals** : The blood vessels of the stomach dilate just after meals. This stimulates the secretion of enzymes, and thus helps digestion. If work requiring any kind of physical or mental exertion is taken up just after a meal, blood will be diverted from the stomach to other parts of the body like the hand, feet or brain, slowing down digestion.

(9) **Do not take any food while suffering from fever or any other ailment** : This is essential. It is a fact that we never do feel hungry when we are indisposed, and actually feel averse to taking any food. During an illness, the secretion of digestive juices is greatly reduced. As a result, the digestive processes are almost at a standstill.

(10) **Eat only one meal, or take only fruits, one day every week** : Giving occasional rest to the stomach is as necessary as giving it its usual assignment of digestion, for maintaining its efficiency. Moreover, when the body is not occupied in the task of digestion, it is free to tackle the poisons that have been accumulated in it.

7. JUICE DIET

Alkali-genic foods, as has been explained in Chapter 6, extract the toxic substances accumulated in the cells of the body and help in their elimination. And this is why such foods are considered to be purifying foods.

Even a healthy person derives benefit by keeping to an alkali-genic diet rich in minerals. Such a diet is all the more necessary in sickness. Sickness is rooted in acids accumulated in the body. To neutralise and deactivate these acids, one must take food which can supply plenty of alkalis. This purpose can be better served by a liquid diet.

In fact, for a plentiful supply of alkalis to the body there is nothing that can rival juice diet. Such a diet also provides sufficient vitamins and enzymes that augment the resistive and healing powers of the body.

It may be argued that well-chewed vegetables and fruits can supply all the necessary minerals and vitamins equally well. But this contention is not quite justified. No one can eat enough raw vegetables and fruits, if they have to be thoroughly chewed. For instance, one can chomp down a carrot or two at a time, no more. But it would be quite easy to drink the juice of eight or ten carrots. It must also be remembered that even if fruits and vegetables are well chewed, a large amount of fibres and woody particles will reach the stomach, loading the stomach and slowing down digestion. In short, when the digestive system is not to be overburdened, and at the same time fasting is not desirable for some reason, a juice diet, consisting of juices of vegetables and fruits becomes essential.

The juices must always be consumed while fresh. This is especially important when the purpose is that of healing or prevention of disease. The vitamins in raw uncooked foods are very sensitive to the oxygen of the air. If carrots, for example, are cut or shredded and then left for some time, most of their vitamin A content gets destroyed by oxidation, within about 20 to 25 minutes. In the same way, lemons, mosambis, oranges, apples, and similar fruits lose about 50 per cent of their vitamin C content in only one month, during storage. If the vitamins in uncut fruits and vegetables are destroyed so easily, it is obvious that the vitamins in their juices must get destroyed much more quickly. The juices, therefore, must be taken without a moment's delay as soon as they are extracted. The juices must not be gulped down, but sipped slowly, so as to give saliva a chance to mix with them and begin the process of the digestion of the carbohydrates.

Many dieticians believe that fruit and vegetables juices must not be mixed, but must always be taken separately.

Canned or bottled juices are entirely worthless for health, as all the active constituents useful for fighting diseases or promoting health have been destroyed by the processing and prolonged storage. Moreover, harmful chemicals have been added to the juices as preservatives. No one should allow himself to be misguided by the labels declaring that the cans or bottles contain 'fresh juice'. Moreover, most of them are synthetic.

Note : Complete and detailed information about liquid diet of juices of fruits and vegetables is given in the book, 'Juice Diet for Perfect Health' by the same authors.

8. FASTING

Fasting is the weapon of choice that Nature Cure wields in the battle against all acute or severe diseases. And it has proved to be infallible.

Diseases can invade the body only if there is an accumulation of acids and toxic substances in it. The efforts of the body to get rid of these harmful substances are what we deem to be the symptoms of diseases. When the poisons accumulate beyond the normal limits in the body, the body makes strenuous and violent efforts to eliminate them. It is these constructive efforts that are mistakenly regarded as acute diseases. The body concentrates all its energies on the process of healing. In these circumstances, the body has no need for, and does not welcome, food. This results in loss of appetite, and there is a bad taste in the mouth. If food is taken at such a time, the energy of the body gets diverted to the process of digestion. Consequently, the elimination of poisons is stalled, and the disease either intensifies or becomes chronic.

In our country, there has been a tradition of fasting from time immemorial. But these days fasting has become a little difficult. A patient suffering from fever may declare unequivocally that he is not hungry, that he has not the slightest desire for food, and there is a bitter taste in his mouth. But family members, friends and neighbours keep on insisting, *"You must have something to sustain you—tea, coffee, milk, fruit juice, porridge—take whatever you find acceptable. But take something you must. Else you will become weak."* They keep urging things on the patient, and do not rest till he takes something. The patient is thus compelled to eat, despite his complete disinclination. The food remains undigested, adds to the burden on the system, and illness is prolonged. In fact, man is the only animal that continues to eat even when indisposed, and even when he has no appetite. It is an incontrovertible fact that no other animal eats when ill.

Some people are convinced that if they forego even one meal in a day, they will become undernourished and death will snap them up in its jaws. This notion is ridiculous. We would be well advised to remember Dr. Dewey's words : **Food taken in illness nourishes the illness, not the patient.**

A little planning and study before undertaking a fast would be helpful later on. For instance, those who are accustomed to make do occasionally with only one meal a day would find fasting for one or two days quite easy. Similarly, those who are accustomed to fasting for one or two days from time to time will not be deterred or inconvenienced by four or five day's fast–or even more prolonged ones.

Influenza, fever, cold, cough and most other similar diseases are cured by only two to three days' fasting. Where long-standing or chronic diseases are concerned, fasting should be planned with some care and foresight, as longer periods of fasting are necessary. In such cases, one must take light uncooked or liquid diet for three to four days prior to the commencement of the fasting period. This initiates the process of the purification of the blood. Moreover, reserves of vitamins and minerals obtained from the raw foods begin to be built up in the body, which come in useful later during the period of fasting.

It is not possible to estimate beforehand the period of fasting required in cases of long-standing and pernicious disorders. It is, therefore, advisable that fasting for extended periods be supervised by an expert. For really long periods of fasting, it is necessary to check the blood and urine of the patient frequently. If ketones are found to be present in the urine or the amount of urea in the blood is found to exceed 45 mg per cent, termination of the fast becomes imperative.

It is also important to see that fasts are terminated in the proper manner : perhaps more important than the fast itself. The digestive organs have become relaxed during the fast. If discretion is not exercised in the quality and quantity of food after a fast, the inevitable result is that the digestive system is unable to cope with the sudden increase in the intake of food, and the digestive process remains incomplete, leading to the generation of toxic substances. This would be a fresh invitation to disease.

After a day's fasting, only fruit juices should be taken next morning, followed by some fruits during the day, and a chapaty with some boiled vegetables in the evening. Normal diet can be resumed on the third day. After a fast of two days, only fruit juices should be taken on the third day, followed on the fourth day by fruit juice in the morning, fruit during the day, and chapaties with vegetables in the evening. Normal diet can be resumed on the fifth day. In fine, light and liquid diet should be taken after a fast for as many days as the days of fasting.

If this rule is not strictly observed, the fast itself may prove futile, and may even cause harm. Fasting becomes necessary in the first place only because of failure to maintain regularity, propriety and proportion in food habits. If the same irregularity impropriety and thoughtlessness are to be indulged in after a fast as before it, the body can once again become a storehouse of poisons, and therefore subject to the consequent disorders.

Fasting for one day in every ten or twelve days even when one is in good health, purifies the body, and thus can prevent the inception of diseases. *

---

* A complete discussion will be found in the book, 'Efficacy of Fasting' by the same authors.

9. EXERCISE

For maintenance of perfect health, exercise is no less important than diet. The reason why our ancestors were healthier and stronger than we are is that they led comparatively much more strenuous lives. Today's mechanization has set man against any sort of exertion.

Here we give a short account of the salutary effects of exercise on various organs and systems of the body.

(1) **Heart and circulatory system :** Regular exercise makes the heart muscles stronger and more efficient. The heart-beats of an athlete do not increase appreciably even when doing something requiring physical exertion, and revert very soon to the normal rate afterwards. In contrast, even a little exertion sends the pulse rate of a sedentary individual rocketing up, and it takes time for the heart to settle down to its normal rate of beating.

The blood vessels dilate during exercise, and so more blood reaches the muscles. It has been found that during vigorous or rapid exercise, the blood circulation in certain muscles and organs increases 25 to 30 times, thus supplying the muscles and organs with more oxygen and a larger number of red blood corpuscles.

(2) **The respiratory system :** Breathing becomes not only more rapid, but also deeper, thus making increased quantities of oxygen available.

(3) **The digestive system :** The secretion of the digestive juices is stimulated by exercise. Thus digestion becomes more efficient. Exercises also stimulate the intestinal movements (peristalsis), resulting in more effective elimination of wastes.

- (4) **The musculature :** Regular exercise strengthens the muscles, promotes their development and increases their efficiency. Stronger muscles lend better support to the joints.

(5) **The skin :** The pores of the skin open up during exercise. The result is a healthier skin, because of more efficient disposal of impurities and dirty.

(6) **Temperature of the body :** The temperature of the body rises during exercise. This promotes the burning up of the toxic substances in the body.

In short, all the systems of the body derive invaluable benefits from exercise. Each one of us should set aside a minimum period of 30 to 40 minutes every day in the morning for exercise.

Two types of exercises are necessary for perfect health : (1) Yogic āsanas (yogāsanas) and (2) exercises involving rapid movements, such as running or swimming. Yogic āsanas tone up the internal organs of the body by subjecting them to contractions and dilations. Exercises involving rapid movements are beneficial for the heart and the blood vessels.

Yogāsanas : Here we are suggesting an ideal programme of yogic āsanas for the stimulation of all the organs and systems.

(1) **Katimanthana :** Stand erect, planting the feet about a foot or a foot and a half apart. Extend the arms horizontally

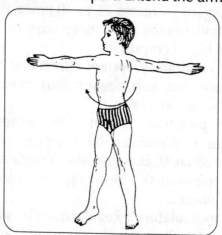

Fig. 9.1 : Katimanthana

outwards at the level of the shoulders. Now, without allowing displacement of the feet, turn the torso round towards the right, and then towards the left.

Repeat the movement 6 times on each side.

Benefits : This āsana keeps the spine flexible by subjecting it to rotatory movement.

(2) **Trikonāsana :** Stand erect, planting the feet a foot or a foot and a half apart. Extend the arms horizontally outward, at the level of the shoulders. Now bend towards the right at the waist, and try to touch the right foot, keeping the left arm vertical in the direction opposite to that of the right arm. Hold this position for some time, and return to the initial position. Execute a similar movement on the left side.

Number of repetitions : Repeat this movement six times on each side.

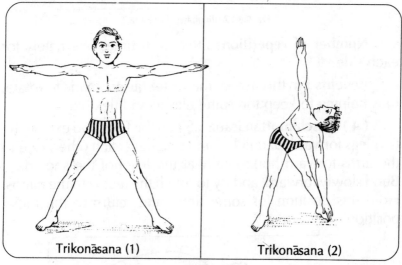

Trikonāsana (1)   Trikonāsana (2)

Fig. 9.2

Benefits : (a) This āsana stretches the spine laterally. (b) The spleen and the liver are strengthened by contractions and dilations.

(3) **Ardhamatsyendrāsana :** Sit down on the floor with the heel of the left foot touching the perineum. Place the right foot on the left of the left knee. Keep holding the big toe on the right foot with the left hand, and with the right forearm placed horizontally in contact with the back, turn the upper part of the torso towards the right. Now carry out the same procedure on the other side, with the right heel at the perineum, the left foot placed on the right of the right knee, etc.

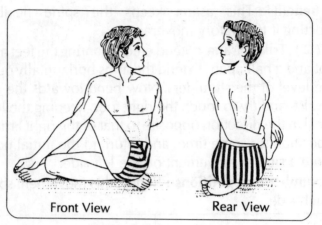

Front View   Rear View

Fig. 9.3 : Ardhamatsyendrāsana

Number of repetitions : Repeat 6 times alternately for each side.

Benefits : In this āsana, the vertebrae are made to rotate, thus helping to keep the spine elastic and flexible.

(4) Paschimottānāsana : Sit on the floor and extend the two legs forward, parallel to and touching each other. Extend the arms forward horizontally at the level of the shoulders. Bend slowly forward, and try to touch the feet with the hands. Hold this position for some time, and return to the initial position.

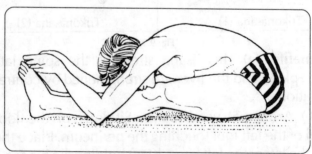

Fig. 9.4 : Paschimottānāsana

Number of repetitions : Repeat the movement six times.

Note : People suffering from hernia must be very careful while performing this āsana This āsana is contra-indicated during pregnancy.

Benefits : (a) This āsana flexes the spine forward. (b) This āsana causes the tightening of the muscles of the organs in the abdomen, thus increasing their efficiency. (c) The muscles of the back become flexible, and the waist becomes less rigid.

(5) **Dhanurāsana :** Lie face down on the floor. Raise the feet by bending the legs at the knees. Stretch the arms backwards to catch hold of the legs slightly above the ankles as shown. Raise the upper part of the torso, and the thighs, away from the floor, leaving only the pelvic region resting on the floor. Hold this position for some time, and return to the initial position.

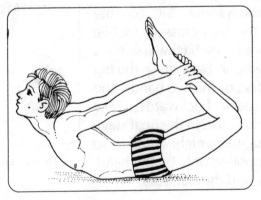

Fig. 9.5 : Dhanurāsana

Number of repetitions : Perform this āsana 3 times.

Benefits : (a) This āsana flexes the spine backwards. (b) The organs in the abdomen are stretched. (c) The muscles of the back and the waist are strengthened.

(6) **Sarvāngāsana :** Lie down face up on the floor. Raise the legs slowly, keeping them straight at the knees. Follow this movement by a gradual raising of the lower parts of the torso. Support the back with the palms, with the elbows resting on the floor. On completion of this movement, only the head, the nape, and the arms from the shoulders to the elbows will rest on the floor, the rest of the body being straight and vertical.

Duration : Hold this position for half a minute in the initial stages. Increase the duration gradually to two minutes.

Note : Those suffering from hypertension or heart ailments must not perform this āsana.

Benefits : (a) The blood flows to the head and the upper part of the torso, nourishing these parts. (b) The thyroid and the parathyroid glands are exercised by compression.

(7) **Matsyāsana :** Sit on the floor with the legs crossed. Incline the torso gradually backwards till it rests on the floor. Now grasp the big toes of the feet by the two hands, and bend the neck backwards. Take deep, slow breaths. In the final stage of the āsana, the weight of the torso is to be supported only by the head, the elbows and the buttocks.

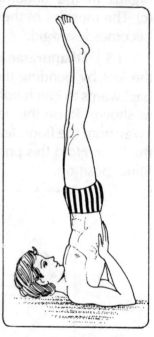

Fig. 9.6 : Sarvāngāsana

Duration : This āsana should be held initially for half a minute, and its duration should be gradually increased to two minutes.

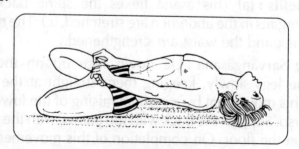

Fig. 9.7 : Matsyāsana

Benefits : (a) The spine becomes flexible and supple. (b) The respiratory system becomes more efficient.

(8) Sheershāsana :

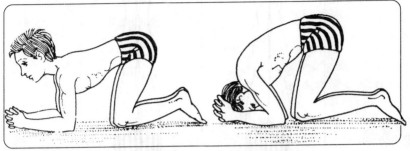

Fig. 9.8 : Sheershāsana (1, 2) : Initial Stages

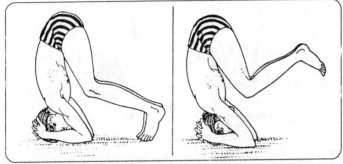

Fig. 9.9 : Sheershāsana (3, 4) : Initial Stages

In this āsana the body has to be inverted and supported on the head. In the beginning, the position should be assumed with somebody's help, or by using a wall for support while

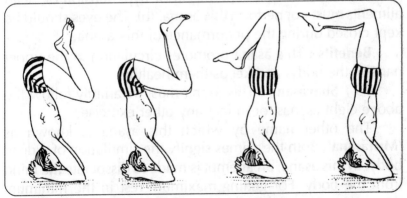

Fig. 9.10. : Sheershāsana (5, 6, 7, 8) : Initial Stages

going through the initial stages. Later on attempt should be made to develop the ability of assuming and holding the position without support or help.

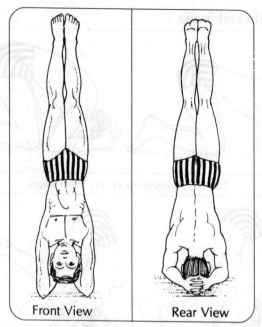

Front View   Rear View

Fig. 9.11 : Final Stage of Sheershāsana

The figures indicate how the position is to be assumed.

Duration : This āsana should be held for half a minute in the beginning, and its duration should be gradually increased to two minutes.

Note : (a) People suffering from hypertension or heart ailments must not perform this āsana. (b) The eyes should be kept closed during the performance of this āsana.

Benefits : This āsana promotes circulation in the upper parts of the body, and keeps them healthy.

(**9**) **Shavāsana :** This āsana must invariably follow the above eight āsanas. or in fact any other exercise.

The other name by which this āsana is known as 'Mritāsana'. Both the names signify the simulation of a dead body. In this āsana, an attempt is made to dissociate the mind from the body. For getting maximum rest in the minimum time, there is nothing better than the Shavāsana. The Shavāsana is universally acknowledged to be ideal for relieving the psychological tensions generated by today's hectic and competitive life.

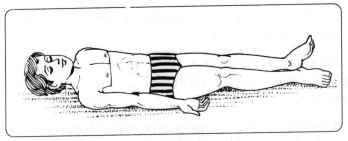

Fig. 9.12 : Shavāsana

The āsana consists of three stages, as described below :

First stage : Lie supine (face up) on the floor without a cushion. Keep the arms and legs relaxed in convenient positions. Now relax the muscles of the body, making a conscious attempt to relax each of the muscles of the body. Begin with the muscles of the legs. Relax and loosen them as much as you can. Then successively relax the muscles of the thighs, lower torso, upper torso, arms, neck and face. To an observer the body should appear completely lifeless.

Second stage : After relaxing all the muscles, turn your attention to your breathing. Inhale extremely slowly, and release the breath equally slowly. Gradually, slow down the breathing action to such an extent that an observer would hardly be able to detect it.

Third stage : The third stage of the Shavāsana is of great importance. But it is somewhat difficult and gaining proficiency in it requires some practice.

The aim in this stage is to greatly slow down the activity of the mind. The ideal state of the mind aimed at in this āsana is a complete cessation of thought; but this state is not attainable by all. However, most of the desired benefit can be obtained if the mind can be induced to hold positive, benign and religious thoughts.

Visualize a religious symbol at the point of the forehead between the two eyebrows, and concentrate the mind on it. Or go on repeating mentally a religious shloka, or a religious aphorism or a name of God. Initially, you will find that the mind wanders off to mundane thoughts. As soon as you become aware that this has happened, concentrate anew on the symbol, or the repetition.

Duration : Holding this āsana for ten to fifteen minutes brings a sense of indescribable peace, restfulness and contentment.

Stimulating exercise, or exercises involving rapid movements : Today the proportion of people suffering from heart ailments is increasing by leaps and bounds. Heart disease has been found to be the root cause of fifty per cent of the deaths in urban areas. Therefore exercises for strengthening the heart– and thus reducing the probability of heart disease– should be undertaken right from childhood. The heart can be strengthened and made more efficient by exercises involving rapid and continuous movements for at least fifteen minutes, so that the rate of heart-beats is increased, and remains high for some time. Exercises serving this purpose include walking at a quick pace, running, cycling and swimming.

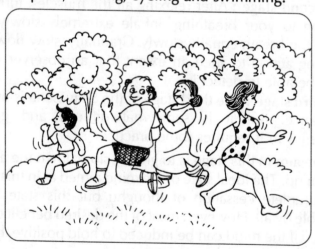

Fig. 9.13

How to implement a programme of exercises : Before adopting a programme of exercises, you must ascertain your normal, resting pulse-rate. Before you get up from bed in the morning, place your fingers on one of the locations indicated by circles in figure 9.14 : (1) on the wrist near the base of the thumb, or (2) on the neck beside the adam's apple.

If you have succeeded in placing your fingers correctly on the arteries, you will be able to feel the pulses as the heart forces the blood through them. Count the number of pulses in one minute, and record it in a table, as shown below :

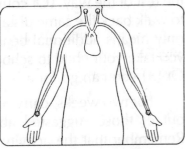

Fig. 9.14

	Date	Pulse-rate per minute
1		
2		

Preserve the paper carefully (or use the space provided in this book to keep a record of your pulse-rate).

Preparatory stage of the programme : It is necessary to start preparations fifteen days prior to embarking on a programme of exercises for increasing the efficiency of the heart. In the preparatory stage you must carry on activities that raise your pulse rate (from normal) to the range described as the 'warm-up zone'.

Find out the pulse-rate in the warm-up zone appropriate to your age from the following table :

Age in years	Warm-up Zone Pulse-rate (per minute)
30 – 34	116 – 126
35 – 39	112 – 122
40 – 44	108 – 118
45 – 49	104 – 114
50 – 54	100 – 110
55 – 59	96 – 106
60 – 64	92 – 102
65 and over	86 – 96

For example, the appropriate pulse rate in the warm-up zone for a person who is 40 – 44 years old is 108 to 118 pulses per minute.

Now find out a way of accommodating a 15 minute period of exercise in your daily routine : (1) Park your car about a mile (1.6 kilometres or so) from your office, and walk the rest of the way. (Of course, this means that you will have to walk back the same distance again in the evening. But this only means additional benefit.) Or (2) you can walk when you take your child to school, or when you go for shopping. Or (3) you can go for a brisk walk in the early morning.

For two weeks, carry on any one activity of your choice out of those suggested above for fifteen minutes a day. Remember that the activity should be brisk enough to raise your pulse rate to the warm-up zone (you will have to determine your pulse-rate to ascertain this) and to maintain it at that rate for some time after the cessation of the activity (for which you will have to determine the pulse rate 5 to 7 minutes after cessation of the activity).

All this is just the preparatory stage of the programme of exercises, not the programme itself. During this stage the muscles and the joints begin to get accustomed to brisk activity, decreasing the possibility of pain in the muscles and joints when the main programme is implemented. Moreover, this stage helps you to make sure that you can undertake a programme of strenuous exercises without any serious inconvenience or danger.

The main programme : The main programme should be embarked upon after the preparatory programme of two weeks.

Find out the desirable pulse-rates in the target zone appropriate to your age from the following table :

Age in years	Target Zone Pulse-rate	Danger Zone Pulse-rate
30–34	136–164	Exceeding 164
35–39	132–160	Exceeding 160
40–44	128–156	Exceeding 156
45–49	124–152	Exceeding 152
50–54	120–146	Exceeding 146
55–59	116–140	Exceeding 140
60–64	112–136	Exceeding 136
65 and over	106–130	Exceeding 130

For instance, the desirable pulse-rate in the target zone for a person who is 40–44 years old is 128 to 156 pulses per minute.

Benefit will accrue to the heart, and its efficiency and endurance will be increased, only if the exercises raise the pulse-rate to the target zone (and the pulse-rate remains higher than normal for a few minutes afterwards).

Look for an activity or an exercise that suits you and that is brisk enough to raise your pulse rate to the target zone. Young men will see that they need exercises involving more rapid movements (running, swimming, etc.) to raise their pulse-rates suitably, whereas older persons would need less strenuous exercises (rapid walking, etc.). Of course, whatever your age, after about a month you will find that you need more rapid movements to raise the pulse-rate to the target zone. This means that the heart has become more efficient, and is able to cope with increase in the oxygen demand of the body with a smaller number of beats.

Recommendations regarding the programme of exercises : The daily period of exercises should be about 30-35 minutes.

(1) The first 5-10 minutes should be spent in activity which raises the pulse-rate to the warm-up zone. During this period,the muscles limber up and the blood vessels begin to dilate.

(2) The next 15-20 minutes should be spent in the main activity which raises the pulse-rate to the target zone.

(3) After these 15-20 minutes of strenuous exercise you must not stop the activity suddenly, but should change over to less strenuous activity for about five minutes. It is highly important that the activity should be gradually slackened, and then stopped. During the period of strenuous activity, the heart pumps the blood rapidly into the arteries. At the same time, due to the pressure on the veins caused by the contraction of the muscles, the blood returns with equal rapidity to the heart. Now, if the activity is stopped suddenly, the contraction of the muscles ceases, but the rate of

heart-beats does not decrease immediately. This results in an accumulation of blood in the limbs, and so the flow of blood to the brain is decreased. This may result in giddiness or even temporary loss of consciousness.

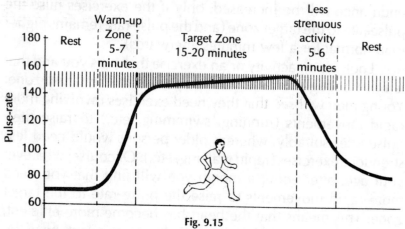

Fig. 9.15

Admittedly, exercise should be rapid and strenuous enough to raise the pulse-rate to the target zone if it is to benefit the heart. But it is necessary to see that the pulse-rate does not exceed the maximum in the target zone (and rise to the danger zone).

After the exercises, it is not advisable to have a hot-water bath, a sauna bath or a steam-bath. There is no objection to a cold-water bath.

Observance of regularity in the programme of exercises is essential. Exercises must be performed daily, or at least every alternate day. Performing them only once or twice a week, or at irregular intervals, cannot yield the desired results, i.e., the efficiency of the heart is not improved.

Determine your resting pulse-rate– before getting up from the bed in the morning– two months after embarking on the programme of exercises as described above. Compare it with the prior rate. The rate will show a dramatic decrease. This is decisive evidence that the efficiency of the heart has improved.

If the heart has been strengthened and made more efficient by a programme of regular exercises involving rapid movements, the possibility of a heart-attack in the declining years of life is almost completely eliminated.

*   *   *   *   *

Two types of exercises have been mentioned in this chapter : (1) Yogic āsanas, and (2) exercises involving rapid movements. Half an hour has to be allotted every day to each of these types. Those for whom it is possible to do this should do the yogāsanas first, and then the latter type of exercises. Those of us who cannot spare so much time daily may devote only half an hour a day to exercise, performing each type of exercise on alternate days.

There is one yogic exercise, 'Sooryanamaskāra', which combines the benefits of both these types of exercises to some extent.

Mode of performing Sooryanamaskāra :

This exercise should be performed preferably in the open, in the mild sunlight of early morning.

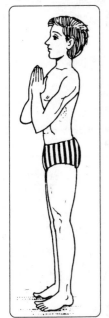 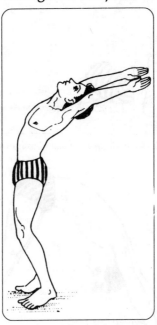 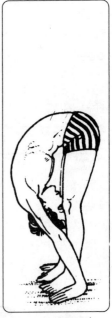

<table>
<tr><td>Fig. 9.16
Position 1 –
Namaskārāsana</td><td>Fig. 9.17
Position 2 –
Parvatāsana</td><td>Fig. 9.18
Position 3 –
Hastapādāsana</td></tr>
</table>

Position 1 (Namaskārāsana) : Stand facing the sun in the posture of namaskāra.

Position 2 (Parvatāsana) : Lift the arms while inhaling deeply, bending the body backwards like a bow.

Position 3 (Hastapādāsana) : Bend forwards while exhaling. Make an attempt to touch the feet with the palms.

Position 4 (Ekpādaprasaraṇāsana) : Inhale deeply again, and at the same time place the palms on the floor, supporting your weight on them, and extend the right leg fully backwards. Bend the neck backwards. In this position, the left knee will be placed centrally between the two arms. On completion of this movement, exhale slowly.

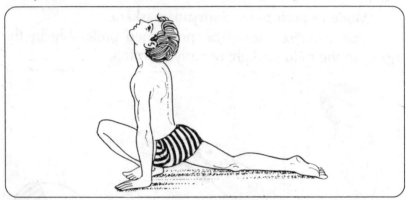

Fig. 9.19 : Position 4 – Ekpādaprasaraṇāsana

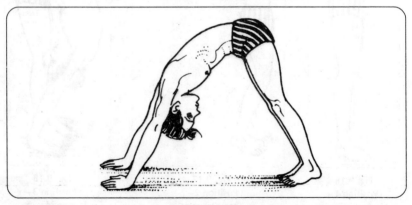

Fig. 9.20 : Position 5 – Bhoodharāsana

Position 5 (Bhoodharāsana) : Extend the left leg also backwards, while inhaling deeply. The body will be bent at the waist in this position, and the weight of the body will be supported by, the palms and the toes.

Position 6 (Ashtāngapranipātāsana) : Now lower the torso while exhaling, till the knees, the chest and the face rest on the floor. The abdomen must not touch the floor.

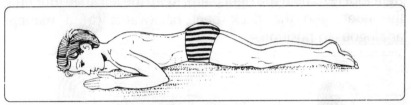

Fig. 9.21 : Position 6 – Ashtāngapranipātāsana

Position 7 (Bhujangāsana) : Bend the torso and the neck backwards while inhaling deeply.

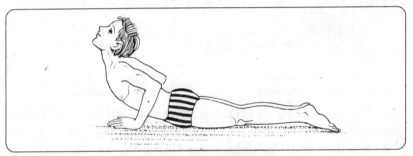

Fig. 9.22 : Position 7 – Bhujangāsana

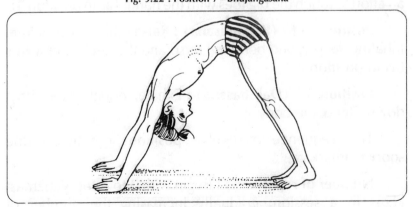

Fi.g 9.23 : Position 8 – Bhoodharāsana

Position 8 (Bhoodharāsana) : Raise the torso while exhaling. Bend the body at the pelvic joints so that the buttocks are raised higher than other parts of the body (as in position 5).

Position 9 (Ekpādaprasaraṇāsana) : Inhale deeply, and at the same time bring the right leg gradually forward, till the right foot rests near the right palm. Keep the left knee touching the floor, and the neck bent backwards (in a manner analogous to position 4).

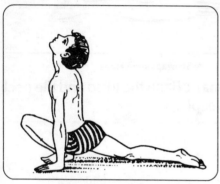

Fig. 9.24 : Position 9–
Expādaprasaranāsana

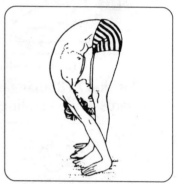

Fig. 9.25 : Position 10–
Hastapādasana

Position 10 (Hastapādāsana) : While exhaling gradually, bring the left leg also forward till the left foot rests near the right foot. Straighten the legs at the knees and make an effort to touch the big toes with the hands (as in position 3).

Position 11 (Parvatāsana) : Raise the arms while inhaling deeply, and bend the torso and the neck backwards (as in position 2).

Position 12 (Dakshāsana) : Exhale, bringing the arms down. Relax the body.

This sequence of twelve positions constitutes one sooryanamaskāra.

Number of repetitions : Begin with 3 to 6 sooryanamas-kāras in a session, gradually increasing the number of repetitions and the speed of each, as stamina builds up.

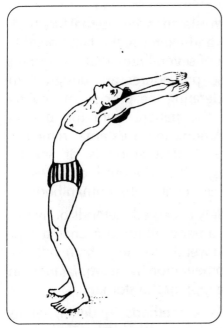

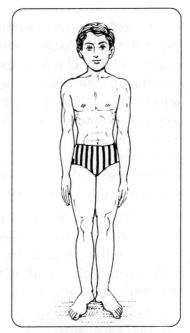

Fig. 9.26 : Position 11 –
Parvatāsana

Fig. 9.27 : Position 12–
Dakshāsana

Note : The benefits of yogasanas as well as rapid exercises can be derived from sooryanamaskāra. If therefore a person cannot for some reason perform other exercises, he should perform sooryanamaskāra 10 to 15 minutes a day. The total time devoted to sooryanamaskāras and the speed of performing them should be progressively increased. If sooryanamaskāras are performed in open air in the mild sunlight of the early morning, one derives the benefits of sun bathing in addition to the benefits of the sooryanamaskāras themselves. (The various benefits of sun-bathing are discussed in detail in Chapter 12.)

10. HYDROTHERAPY

In addition to the regimen related to the internal functioning of the body such as diet and exercise, the Naturopathic system of healing makes use of several remedial procedures external to the body. These procedures are designed to achieve two aims : (1) accelerating the process of healing and (2) providing relief to the patient from the painful symptoms of the disorder. Among these external remedies prescribed by Nature Cure, hydrotherapy is of special importance. Water is an integral factor of our life processes. Actually water makes up 70 per cent of the human body.

There are numerous widely accepted methods of hydrotherapeutic treatment, chief among which are enema, hip-bath, the full sheet pack, local wet packs, steam-bath, hot foot bath, spinal bath, localised fomentation by steam, *jalaneti* (in the yogic tradition), and irrigation of the stomach.

Before discussing all these methods in detail, let us consider the two common uses of water. These are (1) drinking, and (2) bathing.

Every one must drink at least 5 to 6 glasses of water in a day. Best results are obtained if water is taken on an empty stomach just after getting up and cleaning the teeth, half an hour before each meal, and two hours after each meal. In addition, of course, water can be taken as required when needed. The temperature of the water should preferably be neither too high nor too low. A glass of water with a little lemon juice, taken early in the morning on an empty stomach, is highly beneficial. Magnetised water would be even better. The method of magnetising water is given in detail in Chapter 15. No more than a mouthful or two of water may be taken during a meal if absolutely necessary. No water should be taken for one and a half to two hours after a meal.

It must also be remembered that drinking water in quantities smaller than those indicated above leads to constipation, and has an adverse effect on the functioning of the kidneys.

Bathing has a unique importance in our daily life. A bath washes away the dirt adhering to the body, the skin is rendered clean and glowing, and its pores are opened up, thus facilitating the elimination of the poisons in the body through perspiration. The friction on the body caused by bathing and by drying the body stimulates circulation, and imparts a blissful feeling of freshness. A good scrubbing relieves fatigue. People who perspire too freely should bathe twice a day, as should all of us in summer. Everyone should form a habit of using cold or lukewarm water for bathing. A hot-water bath may be pleasant at the time of bathing, but is likely to generate a feeling of lassitude later, whereas a cold-water bath is stimulating. Those who are in the habit of taking hot-water baths would be well advised to reduce the temperature of their bath water progressively till they find cold-water baths acceptable, tolerable and indeed enjoyable. A sparse use of soap while bathing is recommended. Soap washes away the beneficial oils of the skin, rendering the skin dry and reducing its glow. Frequent baths, with a good scrubbing during baths will be sufficient to keep the skin clean and healthy. Multani clay, cream and turmeric powder may occasionally be used with advantage. A mixture of gram flour and butter milk is also highly beneficial. No one should entertain the (mistaken) notion that the use of expensive perfumed soaps will enhance the beauty of the face and turn us into matinee idols.

Hydrotherapeutic Remedial Procedures :

(1) **Enema :** It is said—with ample justification–that constipation is the mother of a host of major and minor ailments. There is no other way to relieve constipation, and to get rid of the wastes that have accreted in the large intestine, which is as simple, as harmless, as effective and prompt, as the enema. It is difficult to predict exactly when a purgative will take effect; and it is easy to imagine the awkward situations that may arise when the effect manifests itself in unforeseen circumstances at the wrong time and in the wrong place.

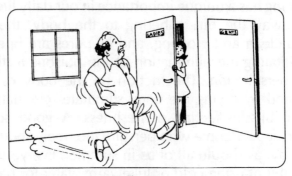

Fig. 10.1

There is an inexpensive apparatus specially designed for convenience in taking enemas. It consists of an enamelled container for water (the fountain syringe, or the enema can), a plastic tube about 5 feet ($1\frac{1}{2}$ metres) in length, a tap for regulating the flow of water, and a catheter, or nozzle. A small bakellite catheter is available, but it would be more advisable to purchase a No. 24 plastic catheter, which is much more convenient.

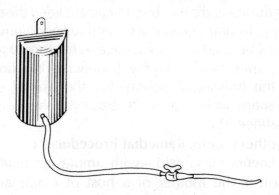

Fig. 10.2 : Equipment for enema

Method : Take a litre and a half or two litres of lukewarm water in the container, and suspend it at a height of about 3 feet (1 metre) from the floor, or place it on a stool of the required height. The end of the catheter should be lubricated with soap or oil. The anus should be similarly lubricated. Let some water escape from the catheter by opening the tap, so as to remove any air bubbles remaining inside.

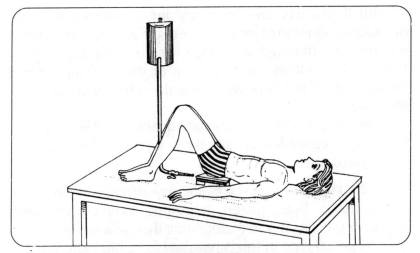

Fig. 10.3 : Method of taking an enema

Lie down flat on the floor as shown in the figure, with the hips slightly higher on a suitable support. Insert 3 to 4 inches (10 cm) of the catheter gently and carefully into the rectum. Now open the tap. The water from the container will begin to flow into the large intestine. If there is reason to suspect anything wrong, stop the flow of water for a time. When all the water has been introduced, remove the catheter. Controi yourself for two to three minutes even if you feel the urgency of elimination, and then visit the lavatory. All the water will be expelled, taking the wastes with it. Do not exert yourself at all to effect the ejection. Sit for a few minutes even after the outflow has ceased. Often an unimaginable quantity of wastes will be eliminated with the help of the enema.

Notes : (a) The enema is much more effective and harmless than purgatives. There are no side effects. The results obtained in 10-11 minutes exceed all hopes.

(b) A daily enema is necessary two or three days prior to, and after the commencement of, a period of fasting or liquid diet regime. In acute diseases, enemas should be taken daily for 2-3 days. In chronic diseases, daily enemas may be necessary for a week or even longer.

(c) Barring exceptional circumstances, hot-water enemas are not advisable.

(d) If enemas are necessary for a number of days, occasional addition of lemon juice to the water for the enema will help the thorough cleaning of the intestines. Except for lemon juice, nothing such as soap or similar things should ever be added to the water. The soda in the soap harms the intestines.

(e) People who take sufficient quantities of fibrous foods like fruits, vegetables, etc., or those who exercise regularly, rarely need enemas.

(2) **Hip-bath :** Hip-baths are very effective in stimulating the stomach, liver, spleen, intestines, kidneys and other digestive organs, and in maintaining their efficiency.

A special type of tub is required for a hip-bath. If that is not available, the oval tubs used for collecting the used plates in parties etc. also serve satisfactorily. Normally the tub for a hip-bath should be about 30 inches (75 cms) long and 20–22 inches (50 cms) wide.

Method : Fill the tub with lukewarm water to a depth of 8-10 inches (20-25 cms). Drink a glass of warm water, and sit in the tub with the abdomen and part of the thighs submerged in the water, and the upper trunk and the legs outside the tub. Keep massaging the abdomen with some pressure, using a thick coarse towel or napkin.

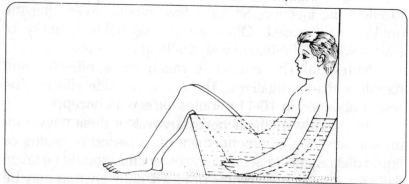

Fig. 10.4 : Hip-bath

The bath may be continued for ten to fifteen minutes in winter, and 20 to 30 minutes in summer. Dry yourself thoroughly after a hip-bath; a few exercises meant for toning up the abdominal organs may be performed.

Notes : (1) A hip-bath should always be taken on an empty stomach.

(2) No food should be taken for half an hour after a hip-bath.

(3) If suffering from abdominal pains, menstrual disorders or premature menopause, hot-water hip-baths are advised. While taking a hot-water hip-bath, a napkin wetted with cold water should be placed on the scalp. Alternate cold and hot hip-baths may prove beneficial in the disorders mentioned. Two tubs should be placed side by side for this purpose, and two minutes should be spent in each tub alternately.

(3) **Full sheet pack** : This is a very effective means of eliminating the toxins in the body through perspiration.

A cotton sheet about 7 to 8 feet long and about four feet wide ($2\frac{1}{2}$ metres × $1\frac{1}{4}$ metres), one or two woollen blankets, and a napkin are required for the full sheet wet pack.

Method : Spread the blankets on the floor. Spread the sheet over them after wetting it with cold water and wringing it. Drink a glass of warm water, and lie down face up on the sheet in the nude, with the arms along the sides of the body. The head should lie outside the sheet. Get someone to wrap the sheet tightly around the body. The blankets must then be wrapped similarly around the body. The napkin should be wrung in cold water and wrapped around the scalp.

You may feel cold for a short time when wrapped up in this way, but soon the pack will begin to be warmed by the body heat. In 15 to 20 minutes you will begin to perspire freely. The perspiration will be soaked up by the sheet. The pack should be removed after 25 to 30 minutes and the body wiped with a piece of wet cloth. Large amounts of poisons in the body are eliminated through the perspiration. This can be confirmed by smelling the sheet.

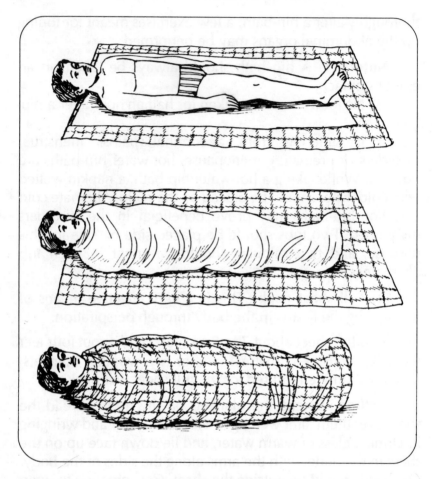

Fig. 10.5 : The full sheet pack

Notes : (1) The principal effect of the full sheet pack is the elimination of the toxic substances in the body through perspiration. If there is a fever, the pack will bring the temperature down by eliminating the poisons. But the pack should not be employed in the initial stages of the fever when the patient is feeling cold, or is shivering.

(2) The cloth used for the pack must be washed thoroughly, and dried, before using it again.

(3) Local wet packs for the chest, abdomen, genitals or the arms and legs may be applied if necessary. The genital wet pack is also called the 'T Pack'.

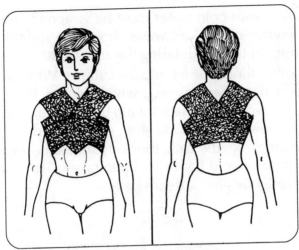

Fig. 10.6 : The chest pack

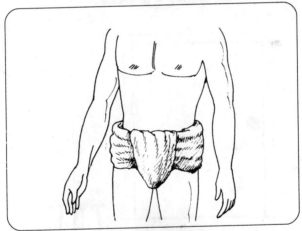

Fig. 10.7 : The genital pack

(4) Steam-bath : This is another universally employed and useful method for the elimination of poisons from the body by inducing profuse perspiration. A specially designed cabinet or steam box is necessary for the steam bath. It can be purchased for personal use, or can even be constructed at home.

Method : This bath is to be taken when the stomach is empty. The patient must drink a glass of warm water and sit down in the cabinet with minimum or no clothing. A small towel wetted with cold water must be wrapped around the head to keep it cool. Cold water should be sprinkled from time to time on the head during the steam-bath. Now steam from the kettle should be let into the cabinet. When sufficient perspiration has been formed, which would be in about fifteen minutes or so, the bath should be discontinued. Excess should be avoided and moderation exercised in this matter. After emerging from the bath, the body should be wiped with a wet cloth, or a cold bath should be taken. The body feels light and sprightly after a steam-bath.

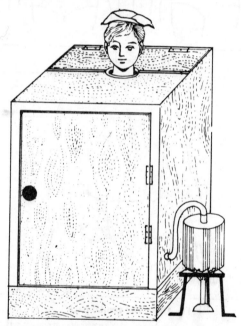

Fig. 10.8 : The steam-bath

Notes : (a) Very weak patients, pregnant women, and patients suffering from heart ailments or from abnormally high or low blood pressure must not take steam-baths.

(b) Normally a steam-bath is advisable once a week. Obese persons may take it twice a week with advantage.

(c) If a feeling of giddiness is experienced during a steam-bath, the bath should be terminated at once. The head should be washed with cold water and bed rest taken for some time, till one feels well again.

(d) Some physicians use a steam-bath to bring down the temperature in fevers. This is totally unjustified.

(e) This is an infallible method of increasing the metabolic rate and reducing weight.

(f) For the purpose of elimination of poisons from the body, the full sheet pack is considered to be of greater utility than the steam-bath.

(5) Hot foot bath : The hot foot bath is an effective means of reducing congestion of blood or water in the upper parts of the body.

Fairly hot water, which should not be hot enough to cause pain or serious discomfort, should be used for the hot foot bath. Hot water sufficient to fill about three quarters of a large bucket, a woollen blanket and a napkin are required for the hot foot bath.

Method : Place the bucket of hot water in front of a chair. Drink a glass of warm water and sit on the chair with absolutely minimum clothing. Immerse both feet in the hot water. Wrap the blanket around the body and place a napkin wrung out in cold water on the scalp. If it is not possible

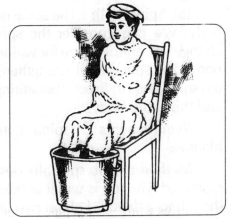

Fig. 10.9 : The hot foot bath

to immerse both the feet in water at the same time, immerse them alternately one at a time. After a time, it should be possible to immerse both of them. In 15 to 20 minutes you will start perspiring. When a fair amount of perspiration has been formed, the bath can be terminated. Cold water should be sprinkled from time to time on the napkin placed on the head. Ladies should normally keep the hair dry (unoiled) while taking the hot foot bath. Alter the bath, the body must be wiped with a cold wet cloth, and one should lie down in bed for 5 to 10 minutes.

Notes : (1) This bath causes plenty of blood to rush to the feet. So there is no reason to worry if the feet remain red for 10 to 15 minutes after the hot foot bath.

(2) If sufficient perspiration is not induced in the expected time, take the feet out of the bucket, and pour 3 to 4 glasses of boiling water into the bucket. The higher temperature of water will now have the desired effect.

(3) The blood pressure decreases during the course of the bath. A feeling of giddiness therefore may ensue. This feeling will pass away on resting for a few minutes. But as a precautionary measure, very weak persons, pregnant women and patients with abnormal blood pressure should avoid taking hot foot baths.

(6) Spinal bath : The spine is a very important part of the body. We can consider the spinal column to be an 'exchange', a control centre for various messages to and from the body. The spinal bath strengthens, stimulates and nourishes the spine, thus indirectly benefiting the whole nervous system and the entire body.

Requirements : A spinal bath tub, a bath towel and a blanket.

Method : A tub specially designed for the spinal bath is marketed. The tub is wider at the top than at the bottom. Fill the tub to a depth of about two inches (5 cms). Lie down in the tub with the arms and the legs outside the tub. In this position, the entire spinal column with the exception of two or three vertebrae of the neck will be under the water level. Wet the bath towel, fold it lengthwise, and place it as a support for the neck and the head on the slanting wall of the tub. When the head is allowed to rest on the towel, the whole spine will

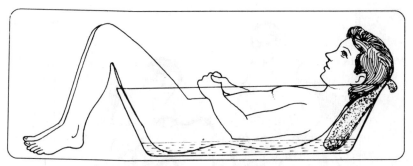

Fig. 10.10 : The spinal bath

come in contact with water. After taking up this position, cover the whole body except the head with a blanket, to protect the body from the outside draughts. The bath should last for about 10 to 15 minutes in winter, and 15 to 20 minutes in summer. There is no objection to wearing a pair of shorts during a spinal bath.

Note : If a suitable tub is not available, a spinal bath can still be taken, on the floor. A towel is wetted in cold water and folded lengthwise to form a 6 to 7 inch (15 cms) wide band. Spread this band on the floor and lie down on it in such a way that the towel is in contact with entire spine. The towel can be folded to a greater thickness under the neck. Then the body should be covered with a blanket as directed.

(7) **Wet or dry fomentation with hot water :** Fomentation is very useful for relief of localised pain or for improving

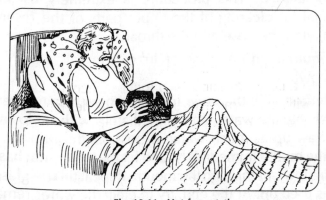

Fig. 10.11 : Hot fomentation

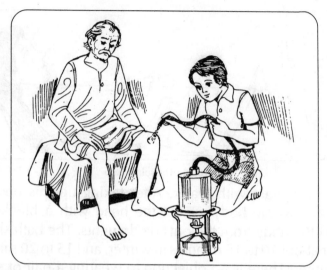

Fig. 10.12 : Fomentation with hot water or steam

the circulation in a part of the body where for some reason the circulation has become sluggish. Covering the painful region with cloth dipped in hot water, subjecting the region to the action of steam from a special kettle, or applying heat by means of a hot-water bag or bottle results in sedation of the muscles, improvement in circulation and reduction of swelling. As a consequence, pain is relieved. After the fomentation, the part subjected to the treatment must be wiped with a cloth soaked in cold water.

(8) *Jalaneti :* This procedure is extremely useful and beneficial for clearing of the upper parts of the respiratory system, viz., the nose and the throat.

Requirement : A glass of lukewarm salt water and a small bowl.

Method : Fill the bowl to the brim with salt water. Dip the nose into the water, and immediately, without losing any time, draw up as much water as possible through the nose. Open the mouth immediately, and let the water that has been taken in flow out through the mouth. Repeat till the glassful of water is used up. At the end, try to eject the water remaining in the nasal passages by blowing the nose.

Note : A feeling of suffocation is likely to be experienced for the first two or three days. The head may feel heavy and congested. But these discomforts will disappear in two or three days as you become habituated to the procedure.

Some experts recommend a gradual increase in the amount of water. The aim should be to use up half a litre to a litre of salt water in this way. This usually proves beneficial.

The *jalaneti* can be performed at any time of the day. However, the early morning is the most suitable time for it, when we clean the teeth. If the nose gets blocked up due to cold or any other reason, causing a difficulty in breathing, performance of *neti* at the time of going to bed would be preferable. Once you are accustomed to *jalaneti,* if there is no other factor contra-indicating the change, it is permissible to use cold water in place of warm water occasionally for the *jalaneti.*

There are experienced persons who recommend that the water drawn in through the nose should be swallowed. But this is not advisable. In order to prevent the dirt collected in the nose from entering the digestive tract it is better to let the water out through the mouth rather than to swallow it.

Benefits : *Jalaneti* cleans the nose thoroughly. It is an infallible remedy for colds. It relieves headache. It has a salutary effect on the eyes and sharpens vision. Congestion of the nose, *'peenus'* and such other sundry ailments of the nose are other conditions which can be relieved by this procedure.

(9) Irrigation of the stomach (Vomiting as a means of cleaning the stomach) :

>   **Requirements :** About four glasses of warm water containing two teaspoonfuls of salt.

Method : The early morning is the most suitable time for this procedure, but it can be carried out at any other time provided the stomach is empty. Start gulping the salt water mentioned above, without interruption, making every effort to swallow as much of it as you possibly can, forcing the water down your throat, if necessary. It is essential that the water should be ingested continuously, not sip by sip. A stage will be reached when you find it absolutely impossible to take in even one more mouthful of water. You will also experience a feeling of nausea, and retching may start.

Bend down from the waist. Put the two middle fingers deep down your throat. This will at once cause the water to be vomited out. After all the water seems to have come out, try once or twice to induce vomiting again. Most of the water will be regurgitated by this method. The rest of it will be eliminated through the kidneys.

Note : Irrigation of the stomach may be undertaken once or twice a month. In certain diseases many physicians recommend that the irrigation be carried out daily or on alternate days. This, however, is not desirable, because elimination of the residual salt water puts a great strain on the kidneys.

Benefits : Most physicians believe that disturbances of digestion, and especially disturbances of the functions of the stomach, are at the root of all disorders. Vomiting clears the aesophagus and the stomach. It relieves acidity, dyspeptic belching, asthma and many other ailments. Occasional irrigation of the stomach prevents such disorders.

(10) Inhalation of salt-water vapour (steam) :

Requirements : About four glasses of salt-water in a large vessel, a large blanket, and wet cloth for wiping perspiration.

Method : Place the salt-water vessel on a stove. When the water comes to a boil, place the vessel on the floor and sit down beside it. You should be wearing the minimum possible clothing. Cover your body and the vessel with a blanket like a tent. Keep your eyes closed and inhale the steam deeply. Lean over the vessel so as to let the vapour warm your face, the inside of the mouth, the nasal passages, and even the chest. There will be profuse perspiration in 5 or 7 minutes.

Afterwards wipe the parts that have been exposed to the steam with a piece of cloth wrung in cold water.

Benefits : Inhalation of steam is an unfailing remedy for colds. It is also useful in all types of disorders of the respiratory system. The fomentation caused by the steam is useful in curing pimples on the face, and relieves cough and asthma. Toothache is also relieved.

Note : Those who are suffering from hypertension or tuberculosis must not take the treatment for more than two or three minutes. Also, they should inhale the steam through the mouth and the nose, but should on no account expose the chest to the vapours.

11. CLAY THERAPY

In the Nature Cure system, the importance of clay or mud as an external therapeutic or a healing agent rivals that of water itself. In fact, the therapeutic benefits derived from the use of clay are very similar to those of hydrotherapy.

Clay is generally used as a paste, to be applied directly as a salve, or in the form of a pack, or as poultice. Usually, clay paste is applied to the abdomen or other regions of the body which exhibit symptoms of the disorder. If necessary, it can be applied to the whole body, or a mud-bath can be taken, in which the entire body with the exception of the head is buried in clay of suitable consistency.

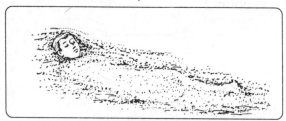

Fig. 11.1 : The mud-bath

The following benefits are derived from mud packs :

(1) **Cooling of the affected part :** The cooling effect of a mud pack is much greater than that of a wet pack. In case of high fever, the temperature can be brought down with the help of a mud pack. Of course, the mud pack will have to be changed frequently till the desired lowering of temperature is effected.

(2) **Absorption of toxins :** Clay has the wonderful and unique property of absorbing toxins from the body. Proof of this power of clay is afforded by the fact that if clay is applied to a boil or a suppurating wound, the pus is quickly drawn out and the wound gets cleaned up.

(3) **Reduction of swelling :** A clay pack will reduce the swelling of any part of the body. This property of clay is well worth trying out by application of clay packs to swollen feet, or other parts.

(4) Relaxation of tension : A clay pack reduces the tension of the muscles and soothes overstimulated nerves.

(5) Relief from pain : Application of clay paste or a mud pack affords immediate relief from localised pain.

Clay of any colour can be used for this purpose, provided it does not contain harmful materials or chemicals. If the clay is highly viscous, some fine sand should be mixed with it. The clay should be sieved so as to remove pebbles, stones and other coarse materials from it. It should then be dried in the sun. When preparing the clay for application as a paste or pack, just enough water should be added to it to give it the consistency of butter. Then it is spread over the affected part, to a thickness of about an inch (2.5 cms). Or it can be spread on a piece of fine cloth like muslin. If clay is to be applied over the eyes, the cloth is essential (as also when the clay is to be applied to the head).

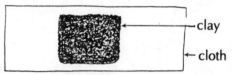

Fig. 11.2 : The clay pack

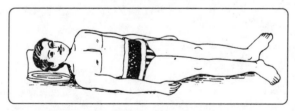

Fig. 11.3 : The abdominal clay pack

If the clay paste or pack is left uncovered, it has a cooling effect on the affected part. But if it is covered well with thick cotton or woollen cloth, generally a warming effect is developed. If, therefore, the aim is to cool the part or reduce the temperature of the body, the clay should be left uncovered. But if a warming effect is desired, it should be covered. Normally, the clay should be taken off after about half an hour, or one hour. If necessary, clay can be applied afresh.

When clay has been used for its cooling effect, the part to which it has been applied should first be wiped clean with a piece of cloth, and then brought to normal temperature by a dry rubbing with the palms. If it has been used for warming the part, the part should be wiped clean with cloth wrung in cold water.

Clay has been found efficacious in fevers, constipation, diarrhoea, gastric, duodenal and intestinal ulcers, bleeding of the uterus, piles, fissures, appendicitis, stomachache, irregularity in menstruation and such other disorders. The beneficial effects of the use of clay on boils, wounds, pain or swellings have been found to exceed all expectations.

————

12. SUN-BATH

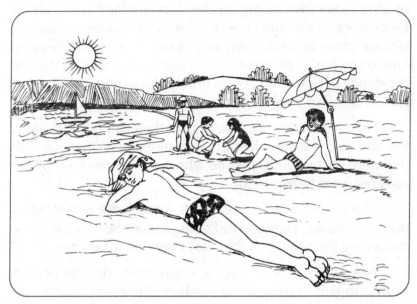

Fig. 12.1

Sunlight is of prime importance for perfect health. Even school textbooks stress this basic fact. But the things we learn from textbooks are usually left behind in the schools. How useful and indeed essential, sunlight is in our life, finds no place in our thoughts. In consequence we invite diseases, generally by wilful neglect of this most healthful gift of nature bestowed freely upon us everywhere, and sometimes by failing to utilise it properly.

The sun showers three types of rays upon us :

(1) Rays of visible (white) light : The white light of the sun is made up of light of seven different colours, as seen in the rainbow. Each colour has its specific effect on the body.

(2) Infra-red rays : These rays impart heat. The warmth of these rays is most welcome in the winter. Moreover, these rays relax and soothe the muscles, reduce swelling and relieve pain.

111

(3) **Ultra-violet rays :** These rays · are of special importance. Vitamin D is produced in the body by the action of ultra-violet rays falling on the skin. Sunlight is in fact the best source of Vitamin D. A deficiency of Vitamin D causes a disease of the bones known as 'rickets'. Dr. Hess of Columbia University has concluded on the basis of his studies that the incidence of rickets increases during the winter in New York city because of the insufficiency of solar irradiation.

Ultra-violet rays are essential for the healthy condition of the skin too. The prevalence of skin diseases is greater among the more sophisticated people who tend to keep their bodies covered from head to foot.

The tendency to disregard the importance of sunlight is on the increase. Ladies avoid going out in the sun for fear of darkening the skin, or if they do, they use sunshades!

Not only the skin, but the entire body derives benefits from sunlight. Exposure to sunlight improves health and augments the resistive powers of the body.

Sunlight helps nourish the muscles. All athletes regularly bask in the sun, as it helps develop the size and strength of the muscles, and increases the proportion of calcium in them, giving them greater endurance. If the skin is deprived of sunlight by keeping it covered, the muscles tend to weaken and degenerate.

Sunlight promotes the proper formation of teeth, speedy growth of hair, and quick and deep breathing. Blood pressure is brought down, and the kidneys become more efficient. By the action of sunlight, skin diseases are cured, blisters are burst and wounds are healed more speedily. Sunlight maintains and even increases the amount of alkali in the blood.

If a pregnant lady takes sun baths regularly, she gets relief from the usual discomforts of pregnancy such as fatigue, backache, nausea, overstimulation (or overexcitement) etc., and lactation in the post-parturition period is also improved.

In short, whether it is a question of the development of a child or of convalescence after a disease has been brought under control, sunlight helps to nourish and strengthen the body.

Pliny, the famous philosopher and physician of the fifteenth century, notes in his book that *'the reason why Rome has been able to develop into a powerful state is that the Romans regularly take sun-baths on their terraces.*

As the survey of the renowned physician Dr. R. T. Trall revealed, even common disorders assume virulent forms among people who work in mines or who for other reasons are deprived of sunlight and have to spend most of their time in the dark. When sufficient sunlight is not available, the proportions of fibrin and red blood corpuscles in the blood decrease, and those of white blood corpuscles and water increase.

Dr. Herbert Shelton states in his book that *"the incidence of cancer is lower in those regions of the world where there is abundant sunshine all the year round. Diseases readily enter the dwellings that sunlight does not. Rickets and tuberculosis take up permanent residence, the incidence of pneumonia increases, and the infant death-rate goes up, in dwellings where darkness reigns. Contagious diseases spread much more quickly in dark and narrow lanes."*

Recommendations regarding sun bathing :

(1) Sun-baths should be preferably taken without any clothes on. But if that is not practicable, minimum possible clothes should be worn.

(2) It is desirable that the head be covered and the eyes closed while taking a sun-bath. Do not cover the face, and **never look directly at the sun.**

(3) The mild sunlight of the morning or the evening has no deleterious effect on the body. It is always beneficial. But it is advisable to avoid exposing the body to the intense sunlight of the midday.

(4) You should begin by exposing the body to the sunlight for 5 to 10 minutes, the anterior parts of the body for half this period and the posterior parts for the other half. Later on, the period of exposure can be gradually increased, as convenient, to about an hour.

(5) A feeling of giddiness, fatigue or discomfort experienced during a sun bath, or a burning sensation in the skin, is an indication of excessive exposure to sunlight.

(6) After sun-bath, a cold-water bath should be taken, or the body wiped with a piece of cloth wrung out in cold water.

13. AIR-BATH

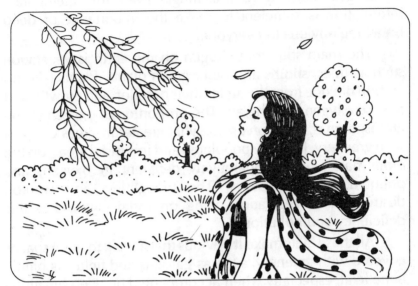

Fig. 13.1

Air is of prime importance for life. One may live for a few days without food or perhaps even without water. But it is impossible to survive even for a minute or two without air.

Oxygen is essential for the process of combustion taking place in all the various cells of the body. We obtain this oxygen from the air. When we inhale, oxygen of the air dissolves in the blood flowing through the fine capillaries in the lungs, and is thus carried to every cell in the body.

Carbon dioxide and other toxic substances are formed in the cells as the end products of combustion and other processes taking place in the cells. Carbon dioxide thus formed dissolves in the blood. When this impure blood carrying carbon dioxide reaches the lungs, carbon dioxide is released into the air present in the lungs, and is exhaled with it.

Thus when we breathe in, oxygen of the air enters the lungs and dissolves in the blood. When we breathe out, carbon dioxide formed in the body is expelled. In short, the blood gets purified in the lungs. Even this elementary information is sufficient to make the importance of deep breathing obvious to everyone.

The main source of oxygen on the earth is vegetation such as trees, shrubs and other green plants. Plants take up carbon dioxide from the air for their nutrition and growth, and release oxygen into the air. The proportion of oxygen in the atmosphere is, therefore, somewhat greater in areas covered with greenery. Densely populated and industrial areas, on the other hand, are comparatively deficient in oxygen, and polluted in other ways. The thoughtless and wanton destruction of vegetation going on today aggravates this deficiency and pollution.

All these facts make it obvious that a walk in open spaces covered with greenery, such as gardens and fields, is highly beneficial, especially when accompanied by deep breathing to ventilate the lungs. The cool breeze of early mornings, being fresh, pure and rich in oxygen, purifies the blood and the body, and fills the mind with cheer and *joie de vivre*. The salubrious effects of fresh air on the body, mind and health are universally recognised.

Some suggestions : (1) Always breathe through the nose. The hair in the nose performs the function of a filter, removing the fine dust particles in the air. Moreover, the air gets warmed up in passing through the nasal passages, which has a salutary effect in the lungs.

(2) Always take deep breaths. The breathing of most city people leading sedentary lives is shallow. The result is that carbon dioxide is not eliminated properly, and toxins consequently accumulate in the body.

(3) Do not cover the face while sleeping.

(4) In winter, protect yourself from the cold with warm coverings as necessary; but keep the windows open.

14. MASSAGE

Massage is another remedial procedure that occupies an important place in Naturopathy. Actually massage has had a very long history, dating back to ancient times. Massage has been used therapeutically for thousands of years in India, China, Greece, Rome, Egypt, etc.

Massage has a very salubrious effect on the organs and systems of the body as detailed below :

(1) **Skin** : The beneficial effects of massage on the skin are unequalled. The pores of the skin are opened up, thus helping of the elimination of poisons from the body through perspiration.

(2) **Muscles** : Massage reduces the tension in the muscles and relieves muscular pain. Strenuous exertion results in the accumulation of lactic acid in the muscles. Massage helps to rid the muscles of this acid and thus imparts a feeling of freshness and vigour.

(3) **Circulation of the blood** : The circulation of the blood in the part being massaged is speeded up, so that the part is supplied with more nutrients, and its healing powers are augmented. The accelerated circulation reduces swelling. There is an increase in the capacity of the blood to carry oxygen and to utilise it effectively.

(4) **Nerves** : Slow and gentle massage with light pressure relieves tension of the nerves and soothes them. Vigorous massage stimulates lax nerves and increases their efficiency.

(5) **The digestive system** : Massaging the abdomen stimulates the digestive system, and promotes better elimination of wastes. The resistive powers of the body are strengthened due to the increase in the efficiency of the liver.

(6) **The urinary system** : Massaging activates the urinary system. As a result the process of elimination of toxic substances from the body through the urine is accelerated by the formation of greater quantities of urine.

(7) **The heart** : Systematic massage will reduce the burden on the heart, and thus increase its efficiency.

Normally dry palms are used for massage; but if the skin is too dry or if the body is excessively weak, wet cloth or soothing oil may be used. Among oils, sesame (til) oil is the best for this purpose. Some people use talcum powder for reducing friction while massaging, but this practice is not desirable, as the pores of the skin get clogged up.

Method : The process should begin with massage of the arms and legs. Next the chest, abdomen, back and buttocks should be massaged, in that order, finishing with the face and the head. Cloth should be used for massaging the back. As far as possible, we should massage ourselves with our own hands so as to combine the benefits of massages with those of exercise also to a certain extent. Those who are too weak to do so may take the help of others.

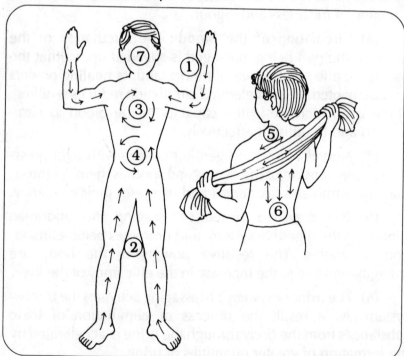

Fig. 14.1 : Recommended directions of movements in massage

The proper directions of movements and sequence recommended for massaging the various parts of the body are indicated in Fig. 14.1.

A massage should preferably be followed by a bath with lukewarm water.

If suffering from high blood pressure, the direction of massaging movements should be reversed, i.e. from head to foot.

Note : Massages are contra-indicated in the following conditions :

(1) In fevers, no massage of any type is recommended.

(2) Pregnant ladies should avoid massaging the abdomen.

(3) Abdominal massages should be avoided in cases of diarrhoea, gastric or duodenal ulcers, appendicitis or tumours in the abdomen.

(4) Massages are generally unadvisable in cases of skin diseases.

15. MAGNETOTHERAPY

The system of Magnetotherapy is gaining in popularity all over the world. The basic tenet of the system is that one remains healthy so long as an equilibrium is maintained in the electromagnetic forces flowing in the body. Illness results from a disturbance of this equilibrium.

Magnets have been in use for centuries for the preservation of beauty and for treatment of certain diseases. There are references to such uses of magnets in ancient writings on therapeutics. But, of course, scientific experiments to test the healing powers of magnets have been undertaken only in recent years.

It has now been established beyond doubt that the electromagnetic waves emitted by magnets affect living organisms. Frequently there are magnetic storms on the surface of the sun. That these magnetic storms have profound effects on the animal life on the earth is now no longer in dispute. Studies undertaken at the Government Hospitals at Hyderabad and Secunderabad have established that during periods of violent magnetic storms on the sun, the incidence of heart attacks increases. The authorities of Indian Air Force also concede that the pilots are more prone to accidents during those periods. The unavoidable inference is that physical and mental disturbances on earth are associated with magnetic storms of the sun. The likelihood of perturbations of the heart, blood vessels, brain and nerves also increases.

Numerous experiments have been performed to determine the effects of artificial—that is, man-made—magnets on plants, animals, and especially, man.

The region in the vicinity of a magnet is known as its 'magnetic field'. If seeds are kept for more than four hours in a magnetic field, they are found to grow more quickly. Precisely similar results are obtained if water that has been subjected to the action of magnets is used to water seeds after they are sown. If flies or mosquitoes are given food that has been 'magnetised' in this manner, they are found to live longer. Magnetic fields have beneficial effects on birds and animals too, birds becoming larger and stronger, cows yielding more milk, horses and bulls becoming more muscular and more powerful. Scientists have had notable success in arresting the growth of cancerous cells in animals, and in some cases even curing cancer, with the help of powerful magnets. Dr. Shiro Saito of the Jikei Medical College of Japan has undertaken large-scale experiments of this nature.

Experiments have been carried out to ascertain the effects of magnets on human beings. It has been demonstrated by many controlled experiments that blood pressure is brought within the normal range, the proportion of red blood corpuscles is increased and that of cholesterol in the blood is reduced by therapeutic use of magnets.

Method of using magnets : Universal agreement has not yet been reached as to the precise method of using magnets therapeutically. Physicians have developed various systems based on their own experiments and experiences, and have found them efficacious in healing.

But it has been firmly established by the experiments carried out so far that no matter what detailed procedure is adopted in using magnets therapeutically, there is a definite and undeniable effect on the entire body. An advantage of this therapy is the total absence of any adverse side effects.

Therapeutic procedures relying on magnetic effects fall into two main classes, based respectively on (1) the Unipolar Method, using either one of the poles, and (2) the Bipolar Method, using both the north and the south pole together, i.e., the method utilizing the entire magnetic field.

Before considering the two methods in detail, it is necessary to acquaint ourselves with the properties and effects of each pole.

Properties of the south pole : (1) The south pole possesses resistive and decelerating powers. (2) It has a cooling and tranquillizing effect. (3) The 'south pole' means 'stop'.

(4) If this pole is kept in ordinary water for some time, the alkalinity of water is increased. In other words, the south pole reduces acidity. (5) It has a contractional effect. (6) It slows down the circulation of blood in the capillaries. (7) It brings infection under control and reduces swelling. (8) It controls and arrests the growth of tumours. (9) Fruits, vegetables, milk, etc. remain fresh for long periods if kept in the field of a south pole.

Properties of the north pole : The north pole possesses properties that are generally opposite to those of the south pole.

(1) It gives warmth and energy and stimulates the physiological reactions. (2) The 'north pole' means 'advance', 'go ahead'. (3) If the north pole is kept in water for some time and the water tested with a pH indicator, it is found to be acidic. Thus it has the effect of reducing alkalinity. (4) It has the property of favouring expansion. (5) It accelerates the circulation of blood in the capillaries. (6) It increases the possibility of infection, as it gives warmth and energy to germs also. It increases swelling. (7) It promotes the growth of both benign and malignant tumours. The tumour, therefore, develops, and may possibly come to a head, burst and heal, or may even spread. (8) When kept in the magnetic field of a north pole, fruits ripen quickly, vegetables begin to decay and milk begins to turn sour.

The south pole proves useful in cases of infection and inflammatory conditions. It is also beneficial in skin diseases, arthritis, infectious conditions, tumours, anxiety, convulsions, eye defects, eye diseases, neuralgia, insomnia, etc.

As the north pole has a stimulating and warmth-giving effect, it proves useful in cases of paralysis, hernia, leucoderma, allopasia, muscular dystrophy, general debility and debility following diseases, fainting, fits, etc.

Dr. A. K Bhattacharya has summarised the effects of both the poles as shown in the following table, in his book 'Magnets and Magnetic Fields'.

Property	South Pole	North Pole
Nature	Cool	Warm
Associated emotion	Love	Hate
Atomic attribute	Proton	Electron
Planets	Mercury, Venus, Moon	Sun, Mars
Elements	Earth, Water	Fire
Colours	Green, Blue, Orange	Red, Yellow
Vāyu (in the Yogic sense)	Prāna, Apāna	Samāna

It is clear from the above facts and discussion that for the treatment of any particular disease or disorder, the use of a single pole is comparatively more logical. Before attempting any magnetotherapeutic procedure, it is absolutely necessary that the specific cause of the disorder be ascertained. If the unipolar method of treatment is to be adopted, a precise diagnosis becomes all the more necessary, as the use of the wrong pole may even prove harmful.

Some magnetotherapists have adopted the bipolar method of treatment. This method too has proved successful in curing certain disorders, though it takes more time to effect cures by this method.

In India, both the chief proponents of magnetotherapy, Dr. Thaker and Dr. Bansal, advocate the bipolar method.

Dr. Albert Ray Davis, the leading American figure in the field of magnetotherapeutic practice and research, as well as Dr. A. K. Bhattacharya and others in India, are staunch supporters of the unipolar method. According to them, the unipolar method may succeed in cases in which the bipolar method has failed to effect a cure.

Nevertheless, if there are reasons or circumstances justifying recourse to the bipolar method, i.e. to the utilization of the entire magnetic field, then this method may be adopted without any misgiving. In cases where both pain and weakness or stiffness occur together, simultaneous treatment with both the poles is definitely advantageous–provided, of course, that there is no infection in the part being treated. The treatment will be more effective if the north pole faces the north and the south pole faces the south. For maintenance of health, daily treatment at the locations of some *chakras* (as specified in Yogic science) with magnets is carried out. Among these, the *swādhisthāna, manipura* and *vishuddha* chakras are subjected to the action of the north pole, and, simultaneously, the *ājnyā* chakra is subjected to the action of the south pole. (See Fig. 15.1.)

Another procedure adopted in magnetotherapy is alternate treatment with the north and the south poles. This method, too, is recommended only when both pain and weakness or stiffness occur together, as indicated above. For treating injuries like cuts and contusions, and vertebral pain, backache, etc., the south pole can be applied for the first 15 to 20 minutes, and then the north pole for the same period. This alternation is similar to the alternate hot-and-cold bath treatment in hydrotherapy.

The specific method of using magnets for treatment depends on the particular disease and the symptoms described by the patient. It is also necessary that there should be frequent consultations between the patient and the therapist, and the method of treatment modified according to the changes noted in the symptoms of the disease.

Magnetotherapy in the maintenance of health : According to Yogic science, there are seven chakras in our body, most of them located in the spine. These are : *Sahasrāra, Ājnyā, Vishuddha, Anāhata, Manipura, Swādhishthān* and *Moolādhāra.*

These seven chakras regulate the electromagnetic forces and energies in the body. Daily stimulation of four of these chakras, viz., the *Vishuddha, Manipura, Swādhishthāna* and *Ājnyā* chakras, for about 15 to 20 minutes by magnets maintains the equilibrium of the electromagnetic forces in the body, thus assisting in the maintenance of health. The following table sets out the pertinent details.

Chakra	Location in the Body	Magnetic Pole
Ājnyā	Midpoint of the forehead	Weak south pole
Vishuddha	On the spine, at the base of the neck	Strong north pole
Manipura	On the spine, exactly behind the navel	Strong north pole
Swādhishthāna	There inches above the lower end of the spine	Strong north pole

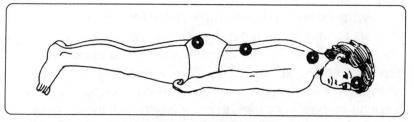

Fig. 15.1 : Locations for placing the magnets on the
body for maintenance of health

Health can also be maintained by drinking 'magnetised' water (i.e. water which has been subjected to the action of the north and the south poles), three to four times a day.

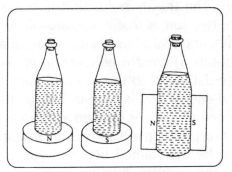

Fig. 15.2 : Method of magnetising water

'Magnetisation' of water for this purpose is effected by keeping magnets in contact with the bottles or glasses filled with water for at least twelve hours. Besides drinking, this magnetised water can be used with advantage for cleaning the eyes, washing wounds and sprinkling on burns.

16. ACUPRESSURE

Today there are several systems that utilize pressure at certain definite points on the body to create specific effects on the internal organs of the body. Among these systems, which include acupressure, acupuncture, shiatsu, zone therapy, reflexology, etc., the oldest and simplest system is that of acupressure.

Acupressure has been employed in the east for thousands of years for maintenance of health, as well as for healing. In China, Japan and Korea, acupuncture and acupressure have been accorded the status of officially recognised therapeutic systems. These systems are being used extensively in the hospitals in those countries. In comparison with those countries, knowledge of these systems can be said to have reached only a minute percentage of the populace in our country.

According to the theory which forms the basis of the acupressure system, the vital energy of the body is made up of two kinds of forces: **yin** (the negative force) and **yang** (the positive force). The theory holds that it is the equilibrium between these two forces that is responsible for the maintenance of health, and that illness is the result of a disturbance of the equilibrium. There are believed to be 14 'meridians' which provide pathways to the yin and yang forces in the body. The vital energy flowing through these 14 pathways is controlled by certain centres located at definite points in the body. By exerting pressure regularly every day at these points, a balance can be maintained between yin and yang, thus strengthening the natural healing powers of the body. Moreover, any specific disease can be cured by applying pressure at the appropriate points on the body.

Acupressure for maintenance of health : The first thing to do is to make sure that there is no pain when pressure is applied at the points indicated below :

(1) The point on the central line of the breast-bone, three to four finger-widths below the lower end of the breast-bone
(2) The points located three finger-widths towards the sides

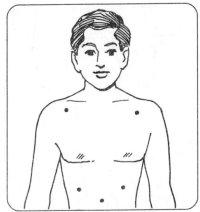

Fig. 16.1 : Points (1), (2), (3)

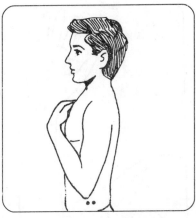

Fig. 16.2 : Points (4), (5)

and about five to six finger-widths above the nipples, between the first and the second ribs (3) The points between the sixth and the seventh ribs, on the same vertical lines as the nipples (4) The points at the ends of the lowest ribs, and (5) the points at the sides of the body, two finger-widths above the upper edge of the hip-bone.

If pressing at any of the above points causes pain, acupressure treatment for two to three minutes at that point is indicated.

Acupressure treatment must then be taken at the points described below :

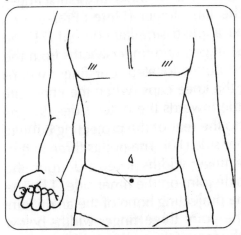

Fig. 16.3 : Point (1)

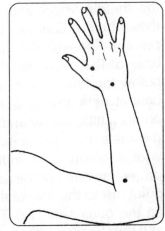

Fig. 16.4 : Points (2), (3), (4), (5)

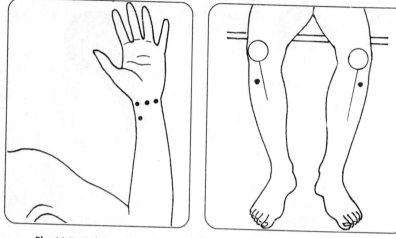

Fig. 16.5 : Points (6), (7)   Fig. 16.6 : Point (8)

The points where acupressure is to be applied: (1) The point on the central line two finger-widths below the navel (2) The point located two finger-widths down the forearm from the outer end of the crease formed on the bend of the elbow when the arm is bent at a right angle (3) The point exactly on the central line on the outer side of the wrist (4) The point in the centre of the fleshy part between the thumb and the first finger (5) The point at the inner lower corner of the nail on the little finger (6) The points on the crease at the base of the palm on the wrist, in line with the first finger, the middle finger and the little finger (**Note :** Pressure on these three points can be applied simultaneously.) (7) The point in line with the first finger, two finger-widths from the base of the palm (8) The points located four finger-widths below the lower edge of the knee caps (when the knees are bent at right angle), a little towards the outer sides (9) The points a little below and to the rear of the projecting bone of the ankle joint on the inner side (10) The points three finger-widths below and four finger-widths foreward from the projecting bone of the ankle joint on the inner side (11) The point just to the fore of the projecting bone of the ankle joint on the outer side (12) The point three finger-widths below and four finger-widths to the fore of the projecting bone of the ankle joint on the outer side (13) The points on the external ear as indicated in Fig. 16.8.

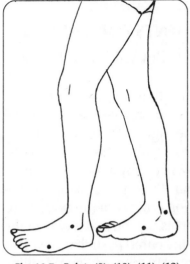

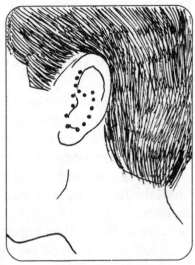

Fig. 16.7 : Points (9), (10), (11), (12)   Fig. 16.8 : Point (13)

The method of applying pressure on the above-mentioned points : Apply deep pressure for 10 seconds with a finger, thumb or any blunt instrument like the stub of a pencil. Release the pressure for 5 seconds. Apply pressure again for 10 seconds and release it for 5 seconds. Repeat this process for 2 to 3 minutes. This treatment should be taken twice a day at every one of the points indicated above.

Here we have shown only those points which are to be treated by acupressure for the limited purpose of maintenance of health, and not for curative application of acupressure.

Note : Acupressure treatment at different specific points is required for the treatment of different diseases. Detailed information in this regard is given in the book 'Be Your Own Doctor with Acupressure' by the same authors.

PART III : NATUROPATHY– IN PRACTICE

17. NATURE CURE TREATMENTS FOR VARIOUS COMMON DISEASES (IN ALPHABETIC ORDER)

It has been mentioned earlier that colds, fevers, pain, inflammation and other similar symptoms indicate an acute stage of a disease. These are the signs of the battle being waged by the body's Vital forces against the accumulated poisons in the body. The renowned physician Dr. Henry Lindlahr has aptly remarked that *"Every acute disease is evidence of the fact that the healing Powers of the body have become active."* If no impediment is placed in the way of the Vital force, the disease gets speedily cured in such cases. This is precisely why it becomes essential to take rest, avoid taking food, and help the Vital force in its task of healing by suitable external remedial procedures. Taking such measures ensures the departure of minor ailments or acute diseases such as colds, fevers, cough, boils, nausea and vomiting, etc., in the short period of two to four days. In fact, by intelligent application of the principles underlying these measures, any one can successfully treat any acute disease, even one which has not been specifically discussed in this book.

If food continues to be taken, medicines continue to be thoughtlessly and recklessly ingested, and other similar liberties continue to be taken with the rules of health, the body drops its efforts to eliminate poisons. The disease then becomes chronic. A chronic disease does not manifest itself in noticeable symptoms in many cases, but keeps consuming the body from within, and it requires longer periods to cure chronic diseases. In treating such diseases it is necessary to begin by taking only raw uncooked vegetable food for a few days, and then proceed to fasting, liquid food regimen, etc., and in addition to take recourse to yogic asanas, magneto-therapy, acupressure and such other external therapeutic measures. If during such a remedial programme there is a sudden intensification of the symptoms, that should be taken as a favourable sign. This is, in fact, a sign of the chronic form of the disease having been converted into the acute form—in other words, a sign of the dormant or suppressed vital healing force of the body having been reactivated. We have seen earlier that an acute disease can be quickly and completely cured. When a chronic disease assumes an acute form, the patient in his ignorance, or under the influence of the alarming assertions of his physician, is led to believe that there has been a relapse, or worse, the disease has been rendered more virulent. This misconception leads him to drop the treatment, and perhaps even lose his faith in Naturopathy. But if he has a clear idea of the real situation as explained above, there is no room for misunderstanding.

Proven and established treatments for some chronic, and common acute disorders are described in this part of the book. But the reader who has studied the first two parts of the book with close attention, and has grasped the basic principles of Nature Cure, will doubtless be able to treat any chronic disease confidently, and successfully.

1. Abdominal pain :
Treatment : (1) Fast for a day or two.

(2) Take a warm-water enema daily for two or three days, and then on alternate days.

(3) Subject the abdomen to fomentation for 5 to 10 minutes and apply a mud pack or a wet pack.

(4) If the pain is caused by gas in the stomach, perform the pavanamuktasana, conducive to the release of the gas via the anal orifice, for 5 to 10 minutes.

(5) After the pain begins to subside, start with liquid diet, then follow it with raw uncooked food, and then gradually resume your daily consumption of cooked food. Continue to take light food for several days.

2. Acidity (Hyperacidity) : Many experts link this condition with emotional tension. Acidity can result also from habitual consumption of excessively spiced or proteinous foods. A burning sensation in the belly and eructations (belches) accompanied by some regurgitation of sour liquid are the main symptoms of acidity. The condition may develop over a period of time into a gastric or duodenal ulcer.

Treatment : (1) Take simple food without too much of spices. Limit the consumption of fried food and sweets.

(2) If suffering from constipation, take appropriate measures to rectify the condition.

(3) Apply a mud pack for 25 to 30 minutes on the abdomen once or twice daily.

(4) Drink water magnetised with the south pole of a magnet four to five times a day.

3. Amenorrhoea : See 'Menstrual disorders'.

4. Anaemia : A low concentration of haemoglobin in the blood is termed anaemia. A person suffering from anaemia appears pale or sallow.

There are three main causes of anaemia.

(i) Loss of blood.

(ii) Reduced production of red blood corpuscles due to loss of activity of the bone marrow (because, for instance, of a deficiency of iron in the body).

(iii) By continual destruction of the red blood corpuscles.

Treatment : (1) Change over to foods rich in iron and Vitamin B. Juice of wheat sprouts (grass), uncooked juices or soups of leafy vegetables, fresh fruit, germinated corn and beans, pulses, etc., are adequate sources of Vitamin B.

(2) Take sun-baths early in the morning or late evening for 15 to 30 minutes. Take deep breaths during the sun baths.

(3) Massage, and wet or dry rubbing are also beneficial in anaemia.

5. Angina : The term angina signifies the severe chest pains caused by insufficient nutrition or oxygen reaching the heart muscles. Mainly it is the process of constriction and hardening of the arteries (arteriosclerosis) that is responsible for the condition. Angina is the precursor of a heart attack.

Treatment : (1) The person suffering from this disorder should reduce the intake of salt and fats in his food. It is also necessary to cut down on consumption of sugar and the use of tobacco. Many experts connect excess of methionine and deficiency of Vitamin B_1 in the body with the constriction of the arteries. As meat is rich in methionine, it is advisable to restrict the amount of meat consumed. Vitamin B is available in quite adequate amounts in raw uncooked vegetables and fruits.

(2) Reduce body weight if it is excessive.

(3) Take measures to control blood pressure.

(4) Perform the shavasana for 10 minutes twice or thrice .a day.

(5) Magnetotherapy is of considerable benefit in cases of angina.

(6) Acupressure is useful in relieving the pain of angina.*

6. Anorexia : See 'Loss of appetite'.

7. Appendicitis : A small appendage at the junction of the small intestine and the large intestine is known as the appendix. This cylindrical organ some three inches (7 to 8 cm) long and about an inch (2.5 cm) in diameter is believed by most experts to be of no use to the body.

The incidence of appendicitis has increased in the present century. A much greater proportion of the more sophisticated urban population suffers from this ailment, while it is rarely found among the backward classes and among the vegetarians. Chronic constipation resulting from the consumption of processed foods and foods without fibrous materials on the one hand, and lack of exercise on the

---

* For detailed information, consult the book 'Prevent Heart Disease and Prolong Life' by the same authors.

other, can be considered to be the main causes of this ailment (Davidson's 'Principles and Practice of Medicine', 1982), Modern medical science believes certain microbes to be responsible for causing appendicitis, but as a matter of fact these microbes are always present in the intestines.

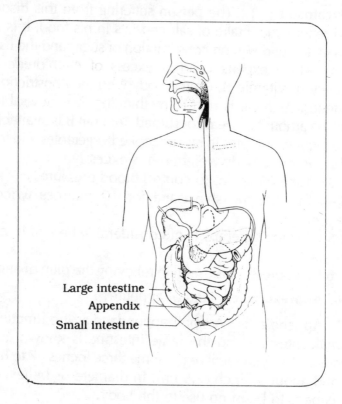

Large intestine
Appendix
Small intestine

Fig. 17.1 : The appendix

Appendicitis begins with pain in the lower abdomen, which gradually shifts to the right. The patient's mouth begins to smell, there is a feeling of nausea and a tendency to vomit, the patient feels feverish and his pulse rate increases. A very grave situation arises if the inflammation of the appendix aggravates to the point at which the appendix bursts. That is why modern medical science favours the outright removal of the appendix by an operation.

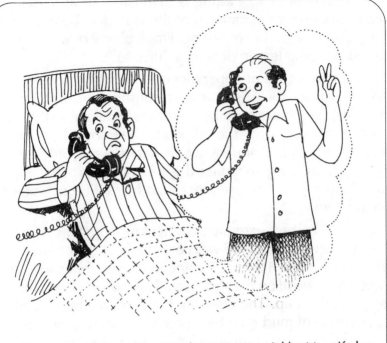

Caller (on the phone) : Doctor, please come quickly. My wife has
        severe pain in the abdomen. I fear it may be appendicitis.
Doctor : Nonsense. I removed your wife's appendix last year. No one
        can have two appendices.
Caller : I agree, doctor. No one can have two appendices. But can't
        one have two wives?

Fig. 17.2

It must be admitted that often the pain on the abdomen or the thigh persists even after the removal of the appendix. On the other hand, in many cases, post-mortem examinations have revealed chronic inflammation of the appendix in patients with no known history of appendicitis. It cannot, therefore, be considered logical to advise removal of the appendix in all cases indiscriminately. In many cases of appendicitis there have been spontaneous cures without any treatment (Frederick Price, M. D., F. R. C. P. – A Textbook of Medicine). In such cases it would not be unreasonable to attribute the cure to the reactivated Vital force.

Treatment : (1) Fasting is mandatory in all cases that show pronounced symptoms of the disorder. Take absolute rest during the period of fasting. Drink plenty of water, occasionally adding lemon or orange juice to it.

(2) In a case of appendicitis, it becomes necessary to take adequate measures against constipation. But for this purpose, purgatives must by no means be taken, as there is a danger of rupturing the appendix thereby. Take warm enemas instead. Frequent warm enemas not only relieve constipation, but also reduce the inflammation of the appendix. Take care not to use more than half a litre of water for each enema.

(3) The best external treatment for appendicitis would be alternate hot and cold wet pack applications on the lower abdomen. After 10 to 15 minutes of this treatment, mud should be spread on the abdomen. The mud must be taken off before it dries up. The alternate hot and cold packs and the application of mud may be repeated as often as needed.

(4) Once the inflammation and the pain diminish, wet packs once or twice a day would be highly beneficial.

(5) To prevent recurrence of appendicitis, once the pain has subsided, fibre-rich diet (fruits, green leafy vegetables, etc.), asanas exercising the abdominal organs, and hip-baths should be continued for a long time.

8. Asthma : Asthma is nothing but the reaction of the body to some poisons accumulated in the body or to the presence of an irritant (an allergen) in the environment. There are two types of asthma : (1) episodic, and (2) chronic. In the first type, there are sudden attacks of asthma late at night or early morning, causing a severe difficulty in breathing. The patient is forced to sit up in the bed, and bends forward in an attempt to ease his breathing. After a time the attack subsides. The patient feels very little discomfort in between attacks. In the second type of asthma, there are no such dramatic symptoms, but the patient has a constant difficulty in breathing. Breathing becomes more laboured whenever the patient has to exert himself, as in strenuous physical labour, walking or climbing stairs.

Treatment : (1) In case of either type of asthma, attention must be paid to diet. A patient of asthma must give up all foods that cause increased secretion of phlegm (कफ in Ayurvedic terminology). The intake of rice, milk, refined wheat flour, pulses, curds, sweets, meat, etc., should be reduced to the minimum. The proportion of raw vegetables and fruit in the daily diet should be increased, whole-wheat chapaties should replace white flour preparations, and the total daily consumption of food should be judiciously limited.

(2) Constipation should be guarded against.

(3) The digestive powers of the body should be stimulated. Yogic asanas for the abdominal organs, early morning walks and cold hip-baths once or twice a day would prove very helpful.

(4) Exercises promoting deep breathing should be performed for ten to twelve minutes daily.

(5) If addicted to smoking, the habit should be given up forthwith.

In case of episodic asthma, appropriate measures must be taken to prevent the recurrence of the attacks. Mental agitation or hard strenuous exercise have been found to bring on attacks. These should, therefore, be avoided. Regular magnetotherapeutic treatment is known to be useful in prevention of attacks of asthma. Certain substances known to precipitate attack of asthma are listed in the following table, with suggestions as to how best to avoid contact with them.

No.	Allergen	Suggested measures to avoid contact
1	Pollen	Keep away from fields and gardens. Keep bedroom windows closed at night.
2	Bed bugs and other small insects	Keep the residence free from dirt and dust. Keep the bedsheets, pillows, etc. clean, and flick them free of adhering dirt every day.
3	Dandruff of animals	Avoid touching dogs, cats, horses, etc.
4	Cotton lint	Use only coir or foam-rubber pillows, mattresses, etc.

No.	Allergen	Suggested measures to avoid contact
5	Fungi	Avoid touching fruit and other things covered with fungi.
6	Certain drugs (e.g. aspirin)	Do not take such drugs.
7	Certain foods	If you notice that particular foods bring on an attack, avoid them.
8	Certain industrial chemicals	Avoid the chemicals, changing your job or occupation if necessary.

In the event of an attack, the following remedial measures are recommended :

(1) Try to avoid mental agitation and keep calm.

(2) Do not open your mouth while exhaling. Let the breath escape through lips only partially opened.

(3) A hot foot bath often causes an attack to subside.

(4) Some experts use wet packs for relief during an attack. The pack may increase the severity of the attack for about 10 minutes, but then a quick relief will follow.

(5) Acupressure treatment may be resorted to. Experiments have shown that pressure at certain points is effective in causing an attack to subside.*

9. Bites and stings : Treat bites as in 'cuts and wounds'. For stings, look up 'stings'. In serious cases such as snakebites, rush the patient to a hospital immediately.

10. Bleeding : Treat as in 'Cuts and wounds'.

11. Blood pressure : See 'High blood pressure.'

12. Boils : Boils can be said to be the external manifestation of poisons that have accumulated in a region of the body. Efforts made to free the whole body from poisons rather than treating boils as a local disorder yield surer and quicker results.

Treatment : (1) Fasting for a day or two does an excellent job of purifying the system. Keep the intestines clean by enemas during the fasting period. The fast should be followed by raw uncooked food for two or three days. Citrous sweet-sour fruits may be taken freely. Intake of salt must be

---

* Detailed information will be found in the book 'Be Your Own Doctor with Acupressure' by the same authors.

greatly restricted. Consumptions of white (refined) wheat flour preparations, sweets and fried foods must be reduced.

(2) Fomentation helps in relieving pain, and in bringing the boil to a head.

(3) When the boil comes to a head, application of wet clay will shorten the time it will take to burst, and the clay will extract the poisons in the boil, thus cleaning it up.

(4) After the boil bursts, application of wet packs assist the process of healing. The pack should be changed every hour.

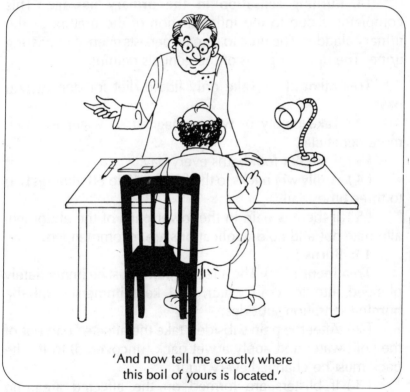

'And now tell me exactly where
this boil of yours is located.'

Fig. 17.3

13. Bronchitis : The wind-pipe (trachea) divides into two branches just below the throat. Inflammation of these branches is known as bronchitis. The main symptoms are cough, fever and excessive formation of phlegm.

Treatment : (1) So long as the acute symptoms persist, no food should be taken. Enemas should be regularly taken to prevent constipation.

(2) Fomentation of the chest followed by a warm wet pack is beneficial in this disorder.

(3) Take steam inhalations twice a day.

(4) Wet packs on the feet also afford quick relief in bronchitis.

(5) It is advisable to take the help of magnetotherapy too.

14. Burning sensation in the urinary passage : This complaint is due to the inflammation of the urethra or the urinary bladder. The urge to urinate persists even after passing urine. The upper regions of the genitals painful.

Treatment : (1) Take only liquid diet for one or two days.

(2) Take plenty of water. Magnetised water is much more beneficial.

(3) Take hot foot-baths every day.

(4) Apply wet packs to the feet for 45 to 60 minutes two to three times daily.

(5) If there is pain in the lower parts of the abdomen, alternate hot and cold applications are recommended.

15. Burns :

Treatment : (1) The affected parts must be immediately plunged into ice-cold water, and kept immersed till the burning sensation subsides.

(2) After the pain subsides, take the affected part out of the cold water and apply a wet pack (uncovered) to it. The pack must be changed every hour.

(3) If blisters are formed on the affected area, no attempt should be made to burst them.

(4) If the patient is suffering from shock as a result of severe burns, and his hands and feet have become cold, you must be cautious in administering the above cooling treatments. Hot-water bags or bottles should be used to keep the hands and feet warm.

(5) Magnetotherapy should be availed of for assistance in bringing about a quicker cure of the parts affected by severe burns.

16. Chest pain : See 'Angina'.

17. Cholera : Cholera is a contagious disease. The onset of the disease is signalled by headache and stomachache, accompanied by vomiting and diarrhoea. Yellowish liquid stools gradually give way to slightly turbid whitish watery stools which in appearance resemble rice water. The body of the patient becomes very cold as a result of frequent and severe loss of fluids. If the disease is not brought under control, the patient loses consciousness, and eventually dies.

Not everyone falls a victim to the disease when there is a cholera epidemic. It does not in any way trouble people whose Vital force is sufficiently strong. The cholera germs are, in fact, found even in the stools of the people nursing the patient, and in the stools of the erstwhile patients who have recovered from cholera, even two months after recovery. In fine, only those people in whose bodies poisons have already accumulated, or in whose intestines wastes have accumulated excessively, are caught in the tentacles of this disease. The body resorts to diarrhoea to flush out the poisons that the germs have produced.

Treatment : (1) The patient should be given a warm enema immediately, as soon as the first symptoms of the disease manifest themselves. The greater the quantity of the water taken up in the enema, the better for the patient. The cholera germs infest the large intestine and the end of the small intestine. It needs plenty of water to flush the germs out. The large quantity of water used in the enema will loosen and remove the wastes adhering to the walls of the intestines. The enema should be repeated every eight to ten hours. Often it is found that the development of the disease is halted by only two or three enemas.

(2) Abstention from taking food is mandatory while diarrhoea persists. During this period the patient should be given plenty of water, preferably water to which salt and juices of lemon or other similar fruits have been added. Magnetised water would also be of great benefit.

(3) Hip-baths and mud packs are of special importance in the treatment of cholera. The patient should be given cold hip-baths every two hours. But his feet must be immersed in hot water while taking the cold hip-bath. Abdominal wet packs should be applied for 20 to 30 minutes between the hip-baths.

(4) In case the patient's body becomes very cold, he should be wrapped up in three or four blankets.

18. Colds : A cold is a very common complaint. Modern medical science has no satisfactory remedy for the common cold, as indicated by the prevalent saying, that 'if a cold is not treated, it takes seven days for it to be cured. But if it is treated, it takes only a week !' But Nature Cure treatment can cure colds in only a day or two. As soon as the attack of a cold is suspected, as indicated by frequent and repeated sneezing, a drink of warm water should be taken, along with a hot foot-bath. This will, in most cases, prevent the cold from developing further. (William Bierman, M. D., and Sidney Licht, M. D. – Physical Medicine in General Practice, 1952)

Treatment : In case a cold does develop in spite of the above precautionary measure, the following treatment should be taken :

(1) Fast should be observed for one or two days. Enemas of warm water, to which a little lemon juice has been added, should be taken during the fasting period.

(2) A person suffering from cold should refrain from eating or drinking anything cold.

(3) Inhalation of steam and a steam facial may be taken to obtain quicker relief.

(4) If suffering from chronic cold, a regimen including purifying alkaligenic food, avoidance of cold dishes and drinks, hip-bath, steam inhalations and body packs should be adopted.

19. Colitis : Colitis is due to old and persistent diarrhoea. Two of its main symptoms are pain in the lower abdomen (i.e. colic), and viscous liquid stools. Debilitating diarrhoea, quickened pulse rate, fluctuating body temperature and a distention of the belly characterise an acute attack of colitis. An unthinking and reckless use of medicines at this stage may result in the disease becoming chronic. The large intestine in such a case loses its suppleness and becomes hard as a pipe, and the patient becomes a victim of restlessness and anaemia.

Treatment : (1) The patient should observe complete fast during the period of persistence of diarrhoea. Water mixed with lemon or orange juice may be taken. Once the diarrhoea is under control, thick buttermilk is of immense benefit.

(2) During and after the fasting period, a daily enema is advisable.

(3) So long as the abdominal pain persists, alternate hot and cold applications for about 10 minutes three or four times a day are recommended. These applications should be followed by abdominal wet packs.

(4) Application of wet clay on the abdomen is also found useful in colitis.

20. Common cold : See 'Colds'.

21. Conjunctivitis : See 'Disorders of the eyes'.

22. Constipation : Constipation is a very common complaint. Naturopathy considers constipation to be the mother of a host of diseases.

A very large number of people can be found, who have not had a natural motion of the bowels for years. When they go to bed, they are more likely to be thinking of their constipation than thinking of their god. They are always troubled by the worry whether the next morning their bowels are going to move. This concern naturally leads them to tablets of purgatives. It is no exaggeration to say that people all over the world spend more money on laxatives and purgatives to relieve their constipation than on all other kinds of medicines taken together. If to the expenses incurred on such remedies we add the expenses on various other remedies of constipation such as *trifala* powder, raisins, *gulkand,* tea, coffee, tobacco, *biris,* cigarettes, etc., the sum total would be astronomical.

Constipation gives rise not only to a feeling of heaviness in the head, gas in the stomach, lethargy, sleeplessness and such other symptoms, but also many more serious diseases with the passage of time.

Causes of constipation : (1) The principal cause is the absence of good regular habits of elimination. People do not keep to regular timings in eating, going to bed, rising in the morning, etc. The natural consequence is that the motions of the bowels cannot occur at fixed hours every day. People who keep to a fixed and regular schedule in their daily activities develop the habit of visiting the toilet at fixed hours – the body gets trained accordingly. However, people living in large joint families, or in chawls or flats with common lavatories, and also those who are on tour or extended travels, cannot visit the toilet as and when they feel the urge. This imposition of unnatural controls on bowel motions may also be responsible for constipation.

(2) Foods without fibrous materials or roughage in them are generally constipating. Insufficient intake of water is another possible cause of constipation.

(3) Lack of exercise, too, is a causative factor. People leading sedentary lives are troubled more frequently by this condition. Perhaps that explains why the prosperous sections of society and the intellectual white collar workers are more prone to disorders of various kinds.

Treatment : (1) The enema is the best and quickest remedy for immediate relief of constipation. It is not possible to predict the exact time when a purgative will take effect, – nor

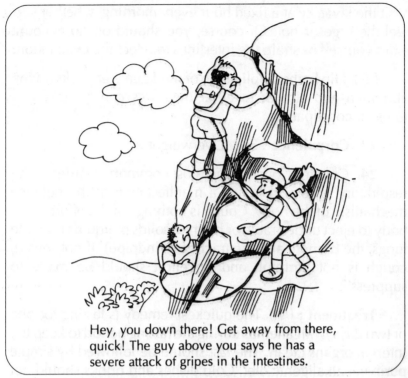

Hey, you down there! Get away from there, quick! The guy above you says he has a severe attack of gripes in the intestines.

Fig. 17.4

the extent of the effect either! – which can result in some funny, and sometimes highly awkward situations.

Moreover, the body becomes habituated to such drugs, lessening their efficacy. They gradually weaken the intestines, too. On the other hand, cold enemas tone up the intestines, and are not habit-forming.

(2) Include foods with flares and roughage in your daily diet. Plenty of raw vegetables, fruits, whole-wheat chapaties etc. should be taken.

(3) Drink a glass of water containing lemon juice every morning. And drink plenty of water during the day.

(4) Yogic asanas toning up the abdominal organs are very useful. And remember, constipation does not trouble people who are physically active.

(5) Try to form regular habits of evacuating the bowels.

Visit the lavatory at a fixed hour every morning, whether you feel the urge or not. Of course, you should on no account exert yourself or strain the intestines to effect the evacuation.

(6) Hip-baths, application of mud and wet packs on the abdomen and similar external measures can be taken to forestall constipation.

23. Corpulence : See 'Overweight'.

24. Cough : Cough is the most common disorder of the respiratory system. It is just a manifestation of the defence mechanism of the body. Cough is nothing but the effort of the body to eject undesirable or harmful solids or liquids from the lungs, the bronchi and the trachea (windpipe). If not severe, cough is not harmful, and no effort should be made to suppress it.

Treatment : (1) The quickest remedy is fasting for one or two days, with enemas during the fasting period to keep the internal organs clean. The fast should be followed by simple purifying alkaligenic diet. Cold dishes and drinks should not be taken.

(2) A wet chest pack has a miraculous effect on coughs. Two or three packs in a day are recommended.

(3) Steam inhalation is an excellent means for getting rid of excess fluids in the lungs.

(4) Deep breathing helps in accelerating the cure of coughs and in preventing a relapse.

25. Cuts and wounds :

Treatment : (1) If there is bleeding, the first step is to try and stanch it. This can be done in the case of the smaller blood vessels and capillaries by pressing with the thumb or fingers, and in the case of the larger blood vessels by applying a tourniquet, using a strip of cloth or a cord. If bleeding continues, the help of a doctor must be sought at once.

(2) After the bleeding has stopped, magnetotherapy should be resorted to for reducing the pain and hastening the process of healing.

(3) The cut or wound should be exposed to solar radiations for 5 to 10 minutes every day.

(4) In serious cases such as wounds due to snake-bites, rush the patient to a hospital immediately.

26. Defects of the eyes : See 'Disorders of the eyes'.

27. Diabetes : This disorder is hereditary to a certain extent. It is the result of the inadequate secretion of the hormone insulin in the body. Diabetes cannot be cured, but can only be controlled. That is why it is important to prevent it, as far as possible. Those who have a history of diabetes in the family should limit the intake of carbohydrates, take regular physical exercises and keep physically active right from childhood.

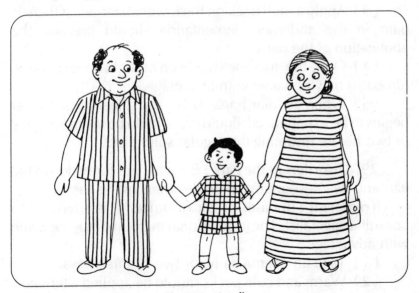

Fig. 17.5 : Heredity

Treatment : (1) The most effective measure in controlling diabetes is a diet with a relatively low proportion of carbohydrates.

(2) Various Yogic asanas, especially those meant for the abdominal organs, as well as exercises, should be performed regularly.

(3) If your weight is excessive, you should endeavour to reduce it.

(4) Magnetotherapy is of great help in the control of diabetes.

28. Diarrhoea :

Treatment : (1) Abstaining from any sort of food is a logical measure in case of diarrhoea. You should drink plenty of water during this period, occasionally adding lemon or orange juice to it. Magnetised water is also very beneficial.

(2) Take an enema everyday till the diarrhoea abates. This advice may sound contrary to common sense, but it has proved of great value in this disorder.

(3) Apply a mud pack on the lower abdomen. If there is pain in the abdomen, fomentation should precede the application of the pack.

(4) Once the diarrhoea has been brought under control, hip-baths may be taken with advantage.

(5) When the diarrhoea abates and a feeling of hunger begins to be experienced, liquid diet should be taken for a day or two before resuming the regular solid diet.

29. Disorders of the ears : Earache, pus formation in the ear, and deafness are the chief disorders of the ears.

Treatment : In cases of ear disorders, it is advisable to consult a specialist. These additional measures may be taken with advantage :

(1) Take an enema daily for two or three days.

(2) Warm and cold packs should be applied alternately to the ear.

(3) Magnetotherapy is beneficial in ear disorders.

(4) Mud paste or a wet pack should be applied to the abdomen to improve general health.

30. Disorders of the eyes : Eyes are the most important organs of the body. If, as they say, there is no sight (दृष्टि), the universe (सृष्टि), does not exist. Truly all wealth and achievements are meaningless if the gift of sight is withheld. Disorders of the eyes are of three types :

.   **(a) General mild disorders :** Irritation, hypersensitivity to light, itching, fatigue, strain, excessive watering of the eyes, etc.

(b) Defects of vision : Short sight (myopia), long sight (hypermetropia), astigmatism, squint, and the sort of long sight that originates at the age of about 42 years, etc.

(c) Diseases of the eye : Cataract, glaucoma, conjunctivitis, etc.

Treatment : (1) In cases of disorders of the eyes, just as in any other disorders, a purifying alkaligenic diet must be adopted. Plenty of raw vegetables and fruit in the diet will supply the necessary amounts of vitamins.

(2) Each one of us must learn the proper ways of using the eyes, and of giving them adequate rest. *

(3) Suitable exercises have been devised for the correction of defective vision. These exercises are indispensable in all cases of defective vision. *

31. Disorders of the liver :

Treatment : (1) Fast for one or two days, taking only lemon juice in water. After that, take liquid diet for a period, and gradually change over to your usual diet. Eliminate fatty foods and alcohol from your daily diet.

(2) Take an enema every day to prevent constipation.

(3) Apply a wet pack to the abdomen after alternate hot and cold applications for 10 to 15 minutes.

(4) A mud pack on the lower abdomen is also very efficacious.

(5) Magnetotherapy also affords relief in disorders of the liver.

---

* For detailed information in this regard, consult the book 'Care of the Eyes' by the same authors.

32. Disorders of the spleen :
Treatment : (1) Fast for one or two days.

(2) Take an enema every day during the period of fasting.
(3) Take a cold hip-bath once or twice a day.
(4) Apply a wet pack on the abdomen or a mud pack on the lower abdomen, after hot and cold applications lasting for 10 to 15 minutes.

33. Dysentery : Treat as in 'Colitis'.

34. Dysmenorrhoea : See 'Menstrual disorders'.

35. Ear disorders : See 'Disorders of the ears'.

36. Enlargement of the prostate :
Treatment : (1) Take a warm enema every day.

(2) Apply alternate cold and hot compresses to the lower abdomen, and then apply a mud pack. This can be repeated two to three times a day.

(3) Magnetotherapy is very beneficial in enlargement of the prostate.

37. Eye disorders : See 'Disorders of the eyes'.

38. Fat, Fatness : See 'Overweight'.

39. Fever : Fever is not a disease in itself, but merely a symptom of some disorder. The toxins in the body get burned up by the high temperature in fevers.

Treatment : Treatment of fevers consists primarily of procedures aimed at purging the body by burning up the poisons and wastes accumulated in the body :

(1) No food should be taken till the fever subsides.

(2) Keep the intestines clean by taking an enema every day.

(3) Apply a mud pack on the lower abdomen two or three times a day.

(4) If the temperature rises very high, apply a cold pack to the forehead, or a full sheet pack on the body. (Do not cover the pack with blankets etc.).

40. Fissures : Fissures are caused directly by constipation. These fissures in the anal opening do not heal easily as they are subjected to abrasion every day while defaecating, and cause a lot of excruciating pain.

Treatment : (1) Fast for two or three days. During this period, daily enemas should be taken, but great care must be exercised while taking them.

(2) Cold hip-baths are beneficial in the treatment of fissures.

(3) Wet clay may be applied locally to reduce the pain and the inflammation.

(4) Magnetotherapy is also helpful in this condition.

41. Flatulence : See 'Gas in the stomach'.

42. Flu : See 'Influenza'.

43. Frigidity : See 'Sexual inadequacy'.

44. Gas : See 'Gas in the stomach'.

45. Gas in the stomach : This is an indication of indigestion or constipation, and usually it is people with sedentary habits that are troubled more frequently by it.

Treatment : (1) Only light, easily digestible food with plenty of fibrous material should be taken. Food should not be taken more than thrice in a day.

(2) Cultivate proper habits of evacuation of the bowels. If prone to constipation, take measures to counter it, taking enemas, if necessary.

(3) Perform Yogic asanas for toning up the abdominal organs.

(4) In this complaint, hip-baths and abdominal mud packs are highly beneficial.

46. Gastric ulcers : Gastric ulcers are generally caused by highly spiced foods, and mental tension.

Treatment : (1) Take simple unspiced food.

(2) Apply a mud pack (uncovered) on the abdomen for half an hour before meals.

(3) Magnetotherapy, especially 'magnetised' water, is very useful in the treatment of gastric ulcers.

47. High blood pressure : Like myopia, diabetes, mental tension and heart disease, high blood pressure, i.e., hypertension, is the consequence of the modern life-style. The incidence of high blood pressure is increasing day by day. High blood pressure has its origin in the hardening of the arteries, and results inevitably in heart disease.

Treatment : (1) Diet plays an important role in regulating the blood pressure. Food containing very small proportions of salt and fats, and rich in vitamin B, vitamin E and magnesium can be considered to be ideal for people with high blood pressure. People suffering from high blood pressure, or hypertension as it is termed, must learn moderation in their eating habits. Only by self-control in the matter of food can the excess weight of the body be reduced. The benefits that non-vegetarian patients suffering from hypertension can derive by giving up meat are beyond imagination.

(2) Shavasana is an unfailing remedy for high blood pressure. Shavasana must be performed for 10 minutes two or three times every day. And if a patient of hypertension adopts, with due precautions, a programme of some of the other asanas (excluding the sarvangasana and the sheersasana), and light exercises, he will benefit in the long run.

(3) Magnetotherapy too has proved efficacious in controlling the blood pressure.

48. Hyperacidity : See 'Acidity'.

49. Hypertension : See 'High blood pressure'.

50. Impotence : Treat as in 'Sexual inadequacy'.

51. Inflammation, or swelling :

Treatment : (1) Fast for a day or two.

(2) Take enemas every day for two or three days.

(3) Take steam fomentation on the inflamed part and then apply a mud pack. Repeat this three to four times a day.

(4) If the feet are swollen, take up a position with the feet on a higher level than the rest of the body, and exercise them for ten minutes or so by wiggling the toes and the feet.

(5) Magnetotherapy is also very beneficial in inflammations of all types.

52. Inflammation of the appendix : See 'Appendicitis'.

53. Inflammation of the throat : See 'Sore throat'.

54. Influenza ('Flu) : Muscular pain, headache, cough, cold and low fever are the main symptoms of influenza.

Treatment : (1) Fast for as long as the acute symptoms persist (one or two days). You may take lemon juice or orange juice with water during the period of the fast. Take complete rest for this period.

(2) Take warm enemas daily for two or three days.

(3) The chest pack is of special importance for getting a quick relief from the disease. Considerable relief from the acute symptoms is obtained by the application of the chest pack even for one hour.

(4) Fomentation of the face with steam can also be taken to reduce the discomfort of the accompanying cold.

55. Insomnia : See 'Sleeplessness'.

56. Irregularity of menstruation : See 'Menstrual disorders'.

57. Jaundice : The disorder in which there is excessive accumulation of a fluid called bilirubin in the body, with consequent yellow coloration of the skin and the mucous membranes, is known as 'Jaundice'. Generally it is caused by an obstruction in the bile duct, which causes the bile to enter the blood stream instead of going into the small intestine (duodenum). The body acquires a yellow colour as a result. Ordinarily, the bile helps the digestion of fats in the small intestine. As a result of the lack of bile in the small intestine caused by the obstruction, fats fail to be digested properly, and the excreta lose their normal colour, appearing whitish because of the absence of bile and the presence of excessive fats.

Symptoms : Retching and vomiting, weakness, loss of appetite, constipation, whitish stools, low fever, yellow coloration of the eyes and urine, pain in the region of the liver, etc., are symptoms of jaundice.

Treatment : (1) Take an enema of plain cold water every morning. Occasionally add lemon juice to the water for the enema. Enema is the best remedy for constipation.

(2) Fast for one or two days. After that, start taking alkaligenic foods. In the beginning, you should rely chiefly on liquid diet or fruits such as juice of citrous fruits, bitter-gourd juice, radish leaf juice, jamuns, etc. Gradually, you can change over to solid food. It must be borne in mind that all fatty foods are taboo for patients of jaundice.

(3) Perform Yogic asanas meant for strengthening the abdominal organs.

(4) Alternate hot and cold applications on the abdomen (especially on the right side) for 10 minutes each should be followed by all abdominal wet pack. It would be of great help if such packs are continued throughout the day.

(5) Abdominal mud packs are also useful in cases of jaundice.

58. Leucorrhoea : Treat in 'Menstrual disorders'.

59. Liver ailments : See 'Disorders of the liver'.

60. Loss of appetite : Loss of appetite (anorexia), or diminished appetite, is a result of sedentary ways of life, indigestion or constipation.

Treatment : (1) Subsist only on liquid diet or fruits for two to three days.

(2) During the period of liquid or fruit diet, take an enema every day.

(3) Drink plenty of water.

(4) Perform Yogic asanas meant to tone up the abdominal organs every morning, and take long walks every evening.

(5) Take a cold hip-bath once a day.

(6) If you are in the habit of taking snacks between the two main meals of the day, give up the habit forthwith.

61. Malaria : The micro-organisms responsible for malaria gain an entry into the body through the stings of mosquitoes. If the Vital force of the person is strong and active, the body quickly destroys these intruders. But if poisons have accumulated in the body and the blood, these micro-organisms thrive in the body, and attack the red blood corpuscles.

An attack of malaria begins with the patient feeling extremely cold, the body shivering and the teeth chattering with cold. Gradually, the temperature mounts, and simultaneously various other symptoms manifest themselves, such as burning of the eyes, headache, and muscular pain. The patient begins to perspire after some time and the fever subsides spontaneously. But at definite regular intervals, the attack repeats itself.

Treatment : The period of respite between two attacks of the fever is ideal for treatment. Take the following remedial measures during such periods :

(1) Give the patient an enema with hot water to which some lemon juice has been added.

(2) Apply the full sheet pack, but keep the hands and feet warm with hot water bags or bottles.

(3) A steam-bath can be given, as an alternative to the full sheet pack. After the steam-bath, the body should be wiped with cloth wrung in hot water.

(4) Alternate hot and cold applications should be administered to the abdomen over the liver.

All these procedures must be completed two hours before the expected time of the next attacks.

As soon as the discomfort preceding an attack is noticed, the patient should drink warm water with lemon juice, take a hot footbath for 15 to 20 minutes, go to bed and cover himself up with blankets. This should prevent the rise of temperature. The aim of the treatment is to see that the attack fails to materialise at the expected time, i.e., is aborted.

If, in spite of all these measures, the temperature does rise, give warm water to the patient and let him rest. If the steps as advised above have been taken, the temperature will hot rise much, and the attack will not last long, the fever subsiding in a very short time. After the temperature has returned to normal, wipe the body of the patient with cloth wrung in hot water.

Experience has shown that by taking the measures mentioned above, in the specified sequence, malaria departs even earlier than has been expected.

In order that there should be no recurrence of malaria, a regimen of purifying alkaligenic foods and magnetised water should be kept up.

62. Menorrhagia (excessive menstrual flow) : See 'Menstrual disorders'.

63. Menstrual disorders : Mentrual disorders include paucity or excess of menstrual flow (amenorrhoea or menorrhagia, regularity of menstruation, and pain (dysmenorrhoea). The nature cure treatment recommended for all these disorders is more or less the same.

Treatment : (1) Take purifying alkaligenic foods, giving pride of place to raw vegetables and fruits. Avoid taking preparations of refined (white) wheat flour, fried preparations and sweets.

(2) Take due care to prevent constipation.

(3) Take a hip-bath every day. In cases of paucity of menstrual flow or painful menstruation, hot or alternate hot and cold hip baths are very useful. In cases of excessive flow or irregularity of menstruation, cold hip-baths must be taken.

(4) The T pack (genital wet pack) is very beneficial in such disorders.

(5) Perform Yogic asanas meant to tone up the abdominal organs.

(6) Magnetotherapy is of great benefit in these disorders.

(7) Other local treatments include fomentation of the lower abdomen (in painful menstruation) or a mud pack (in excessive menstrual flow).

64. Nausea and Vomiting :

Treatment : (1) It is advisable to avoid all kinds of foods if there is vomiting or nausea and retching.

(2) Sucking pieces of ice may help in reducing nausea and retching, and decrease the tendency or urge to vomit.

(3) Those who tend to vomit after every meal should try hot and cold applications on the abdomen half an hour before meals.

65. Nocturnal emissions : Treat as in 'Sexual inadequacy'.

66. Obesity : See 'Overweight'.

67. Overweight* : Overweight or obesity is the result of excessive intake of food and insufficient physical activity or exercise.

Treatment : (1) Restrictions on diet are unavoidable if reduction in weight is desired. Reduce drastically the intake of foods containing high proportions of carbohydrates. Fruits and raw or boiled vegetables should form a major part of your daily diet.

(2) Exercises involving considerable physical exertion must be regularly performed to burn up excess fats in the body.

(3) Magnetotherapy has been found very useful for reduction of weight.

(4) Acupressure treatment is essential for gaining control over the feelings of hunger and the urge to eat.

68. Pain : Today people have become somewhat over-sensitive to, or overconscious of, pain. Of course, it is not at all advisable to ignore pain; but that does not mean that one should rush about looking for analgesic pills the moment there is a twinge of pain.

Treatment : (1) Apply fomentation to the part of the body that is the location of pain.

---

* For detailed information refer the book 'From Fat to Fit' by the same authors.

(2) A wet pack can also be applied to the affected part.

(3) Acupressure is an infallible remedy for pain of any sort.

(4) The use of magnets can also be resorted to for relief from pain.

69. Piles : This is an obstinate disorder that keeps the patient going from one clinic to another, being duped and fleeced by unscrupulous quacks, in his search for relief and cure.

Treatment : (1) If the disorder is a long-standing one, begin by fasting for 3 or 4 days.

(2) Do not allow constipation to persist. For getting relief from constipation, take enemas, exercising extreme care not to cause pain. If it is impossible to take enemas, *isabgul* (white cumin seeds) may be taken for the purpose.

(3) Take a hip-bath twice a day.

(4) Local application of wet clay is beneficial.

(5) Magnetotherapy too is worth a trial in case of pain.

(6) After fasting for 3 to 4 days as directed above, take liquid diet for a time, and then gradually resume solid foods. The food should be such as will soften up the waste products in the intestines. Chapaties of whole-wheat flour (with bran), fruits, cooked leafy vegetables, etc., may be taken freely. Pulses, preparations of refined white flour and other constipating foods should be avoided.

70. Premature ejaculation : Treat as in 'sexual inadequacy'. It is also advisable to control your excitement while engaging in sexual activity.

71. Sexual disorders : These include impotence, nocturnal emissions, premature ejaculation and general sexual inadequacy. Treat as detailed in 'Sexual inadequacy'.

72. Sexual inadequacy : Sexual inadequacy or sexual debility, whether in the form of frigidity, impotence, nocturnal emissions, or premature ejaculation, is more a consequence of emotional and mental problems, though having a physical component.

Treatment : (1) Magnetotherapy is of great help in these disorders.

(2) Cold hip-baths or the spinal bath or spinal wet pack stimulate the nervous system and thus are very useful.

(3) Local treatment includes Mahon baths and the T (or genital) pack.

(4) For augmenting sexual prowess and retaining it to an advanced age, acupressure has proved to be of great value.

73. Skin diseases : Skin diseases are merely the external manifestations of the toxins that have accumulated in the blood and the body. Generally, this important fact is lost sight of or ignored, and skin diseases are treated only externally. That is precisely why skin diseases take so long to cure. But Naturopathic treatment yields very quick results.

Treatment : (1) Only alkaligenic– that is, purifying– foods must be taken in cases of skin diseases. Citrous fruits, i.e., sweet-sour fruits, must be used liberally; and the consumption of spices, fried preparations, sweets and refined wheat flour preparations must be reduced drastically.

(2) Take a cold enema every day or on alternate days.

(3) In the treatment of skin diseases, sunbaths are mandatory. The duration of sunbaths must be gradually increased from about 5 minutes to about 25 to 30 minutes.

(4) To extract the poisons from the body, and in particular those deposited under the skin, steam-baths and whole body wet packs are useful. A steam-baths should be followed the next day by the body pack and vice versa.

(5) For relief in cases of discomforts like skin irritation, pain or itching, or even pus formation, local mud packs or wet packs are highly efficacious.

74. Sinusitis : There are hollow regions in the skull on the sides of the nasal bone. These are known as sinuses. Sinusitis is infection or inflammation in these regions.

Treatment : (1) Fast for one or two days, and keep the intestines clean during the fasting period by taking enemas.

(2) A chest pack yields good results.

(3) Take steam inhalations with facial fomentation by steam.

(4) Magnetotherapy is very beneficial in discomfort caused by sinusitis.

75. Sleeplessness : Sleeplessness is the product of the modern life –style and mental tensions. We find today innumerable persons suffering from sleeplessness, i.e., insomnia. According to available figures, hypnotic drugs worth lacs of rupees are sold every year. But these drugs have their dangers : they produce adverse side effects, and they are habit-forming (addictive).

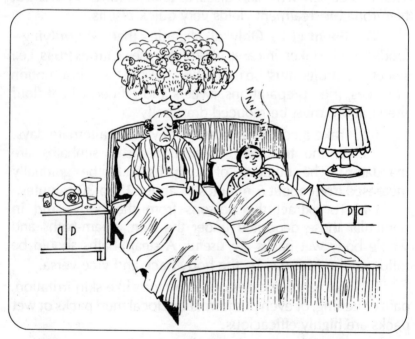

Fig. 17.6

Treatment : (1) Have your evening meal rather early. The meal should consist only of very light and easily digestible food. Avoid foods that, in your experience, cause the formation of gas in your stomach.

(2) Take a long walk of 3 to 4 kilometres after the meal.

(3) Take a hot-water bath before going to bed.

(4) When you go to bed, lie on your back in the bed, place a weak magnet on your forehead with the south pole touching your skin. Perform the shavasana for ten to fifteen minutes.

If sleep eludes you even after these measures, get up and drop all thought of sleeping. Take up a book, and start reading. In a short time, when your eyes become heavy with drowsiness, perform the shavasana again.

76. Sores and abscesses :

Treatment : (1) Expose the sore or abscess every day to sunlight. Gradually increase the time of exposure from 5 minutes in the beginning to about 25 to 30 minutes.

(2) Clean the abscess carefully and apply a mud pack or a wet pack.

(3) Use magnetotherapy to assist quick healing.

77. Sore throat :

Treatment : (1) Fasting for one day and following it up with only liquid diet for one day greatly relieves the soreness of the throat.

(2) Gargle with hot water.

(3) Apply wet packs to the throat and the chest.

(4) Magnetotherapy is very beneficial in cases of sore throat.

78. Spleen disorders : See 'Disorders of the spleen'.

79. Stings (of insects) :

Treatment : (1) If the thorn-like sting of the insect is found to have been left in the skin, remove it by carefully pressing the skin around it and plucking it out.

(2) Apply a mud pack to the location of the sting. Change the pack every hour.

(3) If the sting festers and pus begins to form, treat as in 'sores and abscesses'.

80. Swelling : See 'Inflammation or Swelling'.

81. Tonsilitis : The lymph glands of a special type situated on the upper surface inside the throat are called the tonsils. Inflammation of the tonsils, or tonsilitis as the condition is called, is usually a childhood complaint.

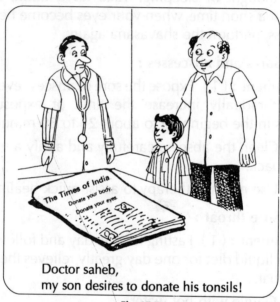

Doctor saheb,
my son desires to donate his tonsils!

Fig. 17.7

There is no part of the body which Nature has produced without any purpose. The tonsils are actually guards standing at the entrances to the respiratory and the digestive systems. There was a time when tonsils were promptly removed by surgeons at the slightest sign of inflammation or infection of the tonsils. But there is no evidence that removal of tonsils prevents cough and colds. On the contrary, respiratory disorders become more frequent, and severe, after removal of tonsils. (Hobar Reimann, M.D.—Treatment in General

Practice, 1948.) It is for this reason that the tendency to remove tonsils has become a little less prevalent these days.

Symptoms : Pain in the throat, a difficulty in swallowing and fever are the chief symptoms of tonsilitis.

Treatment : (1) Avoid taking any food till the acute symptoms are brought under control. But you may take lemon or orange juice in water. After two or three days, begin taking fruit juices, fruits and other alkaligenic foods. Give up fried and spiced preparations, sweets and foods with high carbohydrate content for some days. Enemas during the period of fasting help to prevent constipation.

(2) Gargling with hot water relieves the pain in the throat.

(3) Application of wet clay externally on the throat affords quick relief from the inflammation and soreness.

(4) Wet packs on the throat also yield quite good results in tonsilitis.

(5) After the disorder has been brought under control, walking and taking deep breaths in the open air prove very beneficial.

82. Ulcers : See 'Sores and abscesses'.

83. Urinary disorders : Treat as in 'Burning sensation in the urinary passage'.

84. Varicose veins : Varicose veins are signs of the slowing down of the circulation of blood. This disorder affects people whose work requires them to stand at one place for long periods. Varicose, or swollen, veins are generally seen on the calves of the legs.

Treatment : This disorder requires prolonged treatment.

(1) The first thing to do is to carry out a week long programme of internal cleaning and purification of the body. This will include fasting for one or two days, liquid diet for one or two days, and raw uncooked foods for one or two days, with daily enemas throughout the week. Follow this programme with a regimen of alkaligenic foods.

(2) External treatment consists mainly of cold spinal packs and alternate hot-and-cold hip-baths.

(3) If the veins of the legs have become swollen, perform this exercise three or four times a day : support the legs on pillows at a level higher than that of the rest of the body, and flex the feet at the ankle joints for ten minutes.

(4) Magnetotherapy is also of considerable benefit in the treatment of varicose veins.

85. Vomiting : See 'Nausea and vomiting'.

86. Wounds : See 'Cuts and wounds'.

18. SOME CASE HISTORIES

1. COMMON COLD

Mrs. Niranjana Desai, a neighbour of a relative of mine, came to me early in the morning with her 12 years old son Ramesh.

Ramesh had been suffering from colds for nearly two years. Every 8 to 10 days he used to have an attack of cold. His nose would start itching, he would start sneezing, his eyes would turn red, and watery mucus would start dripping from the nose. Headaches and mild fever would follow. A distant cousin of his father was a doctor. He would administer various drugs such as avil, and the attack would subside for the time being.

But Niranjanabahen was getting fed up with this recurring nuisance. She wanted a permanent solution to the problem. She also mentioned that Ramesh suffered from chronic constipation, and the stools were generally viscous. I examined Ramesh. His nose was watering, the eyes were reddish and the abdomen was hard.

Despite Ramesh's unwillingness, I managed to persuade him to take a warm enema. He was to reach school at nine o'clock. So I let him go, asking him to come back to me in the evening. I instructed Niranjanabahen not to give him his noon meal, but only lemon or orange juice with warm water instead.

When Ramesh came to me at about 5 in the evening, his nose was completely blocked up, his eyes were red, and his head was aching. I gave him steam inhalation as well as facial fomentation with steam, and applied a chest pack. When the pack was removed after an hour and a half, he was able to breathe a little through the nose, and the headache had been reduced in severity. I instructed Niranjanabahen to give Ramesh no solid food that evening, but only warm water and diluted fruit juices, and asked her to bring him back to me next morning.

We followed the same procedure next day. In addition, I gave Niranjanabahen a pair of magnets with medium pole strengths, and told her how to make use of them : (1) for local treatment on the nose twice a day, and (2) to give Ramesh water influenced by the magnets three to four times a day.

When Ramesh was brought to me on the third day, I found that all the symptoms of the cold had disappeared. Niranjanabahen was happy with these results, but was also a little worried that Ramesh had not been allowed food for two whole days. I recommended that he should be given ripe fruits that day, and drew up a schedule of his diet for the next few days, in which leafy vegetables and fruits were the chief items. Directing Niranjanabahen not to give any cold dish or drink to Ramesh for some days, I bade her goodbye.

Nearly seven months have passed since then. Ramesh has not had a single attack of cold so far.

2. CHRONIC ECZEMA

The case of 42 years old Gangaprasad Yadav, a coal merchant, is an interesting one.

Gangaprasad had eczema on the thighs and the nape. The skin of these areas had blackened. There was intolerable itching and burning, and yellowish fluid was oozing out.

Gangaprasad had tried all sorts of medication – allopathic, ayurvedic, unani and homoeopathic – and had used all sorts of ointments, unguents and creams; all to no avail. He had been taking homoeopathic medicines for a year. When all these remedies failed to show an improvement, he sought my advice.

I warned him right in the beginning that prolonged treatment would be necessary, as skin diseases are particularly pernicious and obstinate. Gangaprasad had now lost patience with medication, and he readily agreed, knowing that Nature cure methods do not involve ingestion of lots of drugs.

I gave him a schedule of purifying alkaligenic diet consisting mainly of raw uncooked foods. I strictly enjoined him to discontinue the use of salt, and forbade all fried preparations, sweets, and preparations of refined wheat flour.

I also prescribed these external measures :

(1) He was to take a cold enema every alternate day.

(2) He was to expose the body, and especially the parts affected by the eczema, to the mild sunlight of the early morning. He was to increase the time of the exposure from 5 minutes in the beginning to 30 minutes.

(3) He was to apply wet packs to the affected parts after the noon meal.

Over and above these measures, he was to come to me every day. I gave him steam-baths, and applied full body packs, on alternate days.

On precisely the fifth day of this treatment, his condition worsened. He had fever, and the fluid began to ooze profusely. Gangaprasad was frightened by this turn of events. His family also objected vehemently to the treatment. I calmed Gangaprasad down and explained that all these effects were merely the consequences of the fact that the body had intensified its fight against the disease, so he should have patience. I advised him to fast, taking only water or liquids, and to take rest, till the fever subsided.

The temperature came down to normal in only 36 hours. The external treatment including sunbaths, wet packs, full body sheet packs, steam-baths, etc., was resumed. Gradually, improvement was noted. The fluids stopped oozing. The itching and burning began to decrease, and the area affected by eczema too began to shrink. In about two and a half months, the eczema was cured completely. I recommended oil massages for the darkened skin.

Gangaprasad derived additional windfall benefits from this treatment. He used to be troubled by constipation. Now he had regular motions twice a day. A slight deafness in one ear was also cured. He had been inclined to stoutness, but now his body had acquired almost normal proportions.

3. MENORRHAGIA (EXCESSIVE MENSTRUAL FLOW)

(**Note :** I have been requested by this lady not to publish her name.)

A lady came to me one evening.

This is the gist of her complaints, narrated to me with much embarrassment and shyness.

She was married at the age of 28. She had two issues, a boy and a girl. In compliance with her husband's wishes, she had a metal contraceptive intrauterine device fitted. That is when her troubles began, she began to have copious menstrual flows lasting for ten to twelve days, accompanied by severe pains. It was not surprising, therefore, that her body was pale and sallow, her face lustreless. She complained of gas in the stomach, and of indigestion. She had taken medication for the menorrhagia, and there had been some improvement.

I made out schedules of the ideal diet and suitable yogic asanas for her, with instructions not to perform the asanas during her periods. I also advised her to acquire a tub suitable for hip-baths, and take cold hip-baths every morning. Late in the afternoon she was to apply mud packs over the entire abdomen.

In addition, I showed her the points for the application of acupressure, and the method of taking the treatment. I also gave her magnets of medium strength, and instructed her to use them in the following manner :

(1) Twice a day she was to take magnetotherapeutic treatment by applying the south pole on the perineum, i.e., the region between the genitals and the anus.

(2) She was to drink magnetised water four times a day.

The results of the treatment were gratifying. Within two

months she was completely free from all the troubles connected with the ailment.

4. HIGH BLOOD PRESSURE (HYPERTENSION) AND

CHEST PAINS

Motichand Bhimani is the owner of some power-looms at Bhiwandi near Mumbai.

One of his acquaintances brought him to me.

Motichand was fairly stout, and had been suffering for two years from high blood pressure. A fortnight before he came to me, he had pains in the chest. The local doctor diagnosed it as angina. He also prescribed some medicine for controlling blood pressure.

Two days prior to the visit, the chest pains had recurred. The pain was ameliorated with the help of medication, but it set Motichand thinking. Perhaps something in addition to swallowing medicines ought to be done?

I examined him. He weighed 80 kg. The blood pressure was 135/95 at the time. The abdomen and the bowels were hard.

Motichand was accustomed to bland food. He rarely ate fruit. He used to drink 10 to 12 cups of tea in a day. He had always been suffering from chronic constipation and gas.

I drew up a table of foods with very little salt and plenty of fibrous materials (raw vegetables) for him. I instructed him to perform the shavasana for 10 to 15 minutes twice a day, and also enjoined upon him to bring about certain deep-seated changes in his outlook and general attitudes.

In addition, I gave him a strap with magnets attached to it, to be worn on the wrist. This was for controlling the hypertension. I also showed him the points for acupressure treatment. There was no significant improvement when he came to me again after 15 days of the suggested treatment. His weight was 81 kg and the blood pressure 130/95. I once again explained to him the absolute necessity of reducing his weight, and reduced his allowance of food.

This time Motichand adhered rigidly to the regimen. As a consequence, he noted a gradual improvement in his health. When he visited me again after another month, his weight had gone down to 75 kg and the blood pressure measured 125/90. I recommended a continuation of the same treatment.

I did not hear from him for quite a long time after this. But one morning there was a phone call from him. He reported that the previous evening he had felt giddy, and had consulted the local doctor. The doctor found that Motichand's blood pressure had **fallen** to too **low** a level, and advised him to reduce the dosage of the medicine he was taking for control of his hypertension to *half*!

Motichand offered his thanks to me, and rang off.

For the last ten months, Motichand has had no recurrence of chest pains.

5. CHRONIC CONSTIPATION

48 years old Mavjibhai Vora is a cloth merchant. His life is, therefore, completely sedentary.

Mavjibhai had been suffering from constipation for years. Sometimes he would visit the lavatory after an interval of one and a half days, sometimes after two days, sometimes after the lapse of as many as three days. The stools were invariably viscous and malodorous. Other complaints included gas in the stomach, lack of appetite, bad breath (halitosis) and a feeling of heaviness in the head.

Mavjibhai's face was a picture of despair when he came to me. He had, on his own admission, spent a fortune on laxatives. For some months he had been taking *isabgul* regularly every night, but the results were disappointing.

I inquired about his food habits. His meals used to consist of dal, vegetables, rice and chapaties. He used to have two snacks in the day, consisting of *puries* or *ganthias*.

He had little inclination for raw vegetables, salads or fruits, and he disliked any sort of physical exertion.

I explained to him the importance of fibrous materials and roughage in the diet, and gave him a schedule of daily diet full of vegetables and fruits, and also gave him a table of yogic asanas.

He was to drink a glass of warm water with lemon juice every morning and take a daily morning enema for some days. Even after that period, I advised him to go and sit in the lavatory regularly at a fixed time every day, whether he felt the urge or not.

I also recommended that he should obtain a tub suitable for hip-baths, and take a hip-bath every day, as these baths are particularly useful in cases of constipation.

In addition, I showed him the points for acupressure useful in the treatment of constipation, and gave him a pair of strong magnets to magnetise water. He was to drink magnetised water three to four times a day.

The marvellous efficacy of the treatment was exhibited in just eight days. Mavjibhai considers the cure of his constipation as nothing short of a miracle.

6. HEADACHE

Thirty one years old Vinayak Patil, a resident of Vashi, New Mumbai. had been having headaches for seven years. About once a month, there would be a sudden attack of migraine-like blinding headache, with nausea and vomiting. Analgesics did not help much. Vinayak would be forced to sit or lie down at home all day, with his head pressed between his palms. The headache would not subside until the next morning.

Vinayak had undergone numerous diagnostic tests, including CT Scan, as advised by his family doctor and other consultants. But no cause of the headaches could be determined.

An uncle of Vinayak's had been treated earlier by me, and he advised Vinayak to try Naturopathy. Vinayak could not believe that the simple Naturopathic remedies would work where all other remedies, common and uncommon, had failed. But yielding to the persistence of his uncle, he came to me. Vinayak clarified that he had no other complaints.

I recommended certain changes in his diet, and advised him to give up meat for a time. The diet was to consist mainly of fruits and raw vegetables. I gave him a list of yogic asanas to be performed every morning, before which he was to drink a glass of water with lemon juice. I also advised treatment on the forehead with the south pole of a stall magnet, and acupressure treatment at certain points.

It was quite two months and a half before the next attack of headache occurred. I sent him home with advice to fast till the headache subsided, and to take liquid diet for a day or two after the fasts.

After about five weeks, he had another attack. However, the attack was very mild this time, and subsided after a nap of two hours.

One and a half years have passed since then. Vinayak's headache has not recurred.

7. OBESITY (FATNESS, OVERWEIGHT)

Hasmukh Shah appeared quite agitated and worried when he came to me.

He was very fat, but I avoided mentioning this, and simply asked him the reason of his agitation. It appeared that two months ago, at the instance of his family doctor, he had started on a course of a medicine called 'flabbolin' (Phen-fluramine) for reducing fat. Gradually, his weight had begun to decrease, but so had his sleep as well. It did not occur to him that the loss of sleep was an undesirable side effect of the medicine. During the last four days, he was greatly harassed by various ailments like severe abdominal pains, frequent loose stools, suffocation, parching of the throat and a recurrent thirst. He narrated his troubles to his family doctor on the phone, and the doctor instructed him to stop taking the medicine immediately.

Hasmukhbhai was a gourmand, fond of spicy and tasty foods. That was precisely why he preferred medicines to a change of diet for reducing his weight. But now the dangers and risks associated with the use of medicines were brought home to him. He, therefore, came to me in a state of anxious concern. He weighed 90 kg. Taking his height into account, his weight should have been around 60 kg. Thus his weight was 50% in excess of the accepted norm. I explained to him that gradual reduction in his weight would be safer, and drew up a schedule of diet for him that would supply 800 to 1000 calories per day. As his blood pressure was normal, I felt secure in advising him to jog for a short distance every morning.

A month of this regimen failed to have any appreciable effect on his weight. So I cut down the calories in his diet still further. Another fortnight passed, without any reduction in his weight, I was greatly surprised. It was brought out in our discussion that Hasmukhbhai's fondness for tasty foods had proved too much for him, and even during the period of the treatment, he occasionally indulged this craving. He admitted that he had not been able to adhere to the restrictions imposed by me, under the joint compulsion of his hunger and his craving for tasty foods.

I gave him the following instructions :

(1) Use saccharin in place of sugar.

(2) Eat three or four cucumbers before the noon and the evening meals. He was to cut the cucumbers himself, cutting off a small piece at a time, and proceed to eat it, chewing each piece ten to twelve times. The whole process was to last for ten minutes at least. During the meal, too, he was to chew each morsel ten to twelve times, and follow every four morsels by a few sips of water.

(3) If unable to endure the pangs of hunger between the main meals, he was to eat cucumbers, carrots, radishes, tomatoes and similar vegetable foods only.

(4) Keep notes of all foods taken during the day.

(5) Walk two or three kilometres early in the morning, and also one hour after the evening meal.

(6) Check and record the weight every third day.

I enjoined upon him to observe these rules strictly.

At last, the treatment was successful. Hasmukhbhai's weight began to come down rapidly. As his weight went on decreasing, his enthusiasm and care went on increasing. He kept extending the period of his morning walks. At the end of four months, his weight had been reduced to 65 kg.

②

Fifty-years old Pravinchandra Shah is a Chartered Accountant. His office is located in the prestigious Fort area of Mumbai,

It was during a routine check up of his urine and blood that it was accidentally revealed that he was a diabetic. Pravinbhai was greatly worried. He knew how serious the condition was, as some of the members of his family had fallen victims to this disease before that time.

In addition to being given medicines for the treatment of diabetes, Pravinbhai had been advised to reduce his weight. In his eagerness to reduce, he reduced his intake of food almost to the point of starvation. Within three short days the deleterious effects of this combination of the starvation diet and anti-diabetes drugs became apparent : a feeling of heaviness in the head, giddiness, debility, etc. One day he had a fall in his office due to the giddiness; luckily there was no serious injury.

Frightened at this occurrence, he came to me. It was obvious that he had to reduce his weight. But I advised him to adopt more rational ways of doing so. I urged him to increase his intake of food, and prescribed certain exercises, with a suggestion to come, if at all possible, to my Health Care Centre to perform these exercises. This he agreed to do.

With such supervised regulation of diet and the accompanying exercises, there was no further difficulty in effecting the desired reduction in his weight.

8. ACIDITY (HYPERACIDITY)

Some time ago, I happened to meet a young industrialist. He was greatly bothered by the cut-throat competition in business, shortage of funds, labour problems, etc. The mental tensions occasioned by all these, compounded by irregular and perhaps improper habits of eating and drinking had ultimately induced gastric ulcers.

Changes of diet and antacid tablets did afford him some relief, but that proved only temporary. Occasionally the burning sensation and pain in the stomach would become so acute that he could not even sleep at night. Traces of blood would be found in the stools. He had been reduced to a state of distraction and prostration.

He appealed to me to suggest a remedy for his ailment, if indeed there was any.

I asked him to change over to a simpler diet. I also advised him to drink small quantities of the raw juice of cabbages four or five times a day, consuming in all one half to three quarters of a litre of such juice in a day. He was to take juices of papayas and raw potatoes between the drinks of cabbage juice. I suggested some measures for relieving the mental tension as well.

There was a phone call from him a week later, reporting that he was feeling much better. The cabbage and potato juices were most distasteful to this young gourmet. But as the juices seemed to help him so much, he became more enthusiastic about them, and later on came even to relish them.

After a few days he visited me personally. Nearly all his distressing symptoms had disappeared completely. He was so much impressed by the miraculous curative effects of the liquid diet that he had begun to urge such liquid diet on the other members of his family too.

9. APPENDICITIS

Sheila had been having abdominal pains for about a year. The pain used to be accompanied by nausea and a tendency to vomit. Medicines would give some relief, but the trouble would begin anew after a few days. Ultimately the family doctor came to suspect appendicitis and advised that a surgeon be consulted. A radiograph was taken. The surgeon advised immediate operation, saying that there was absolutely no other remedy. A visit was paid to the hospital with the surgeon's note of recommendation, and the date of the operation was finalised. The operation was scheduled exactly fifteen days later.

But three days later Sheila's father was unexpectedly required to go to his home town. He left instructions that if he could not return by the date of the operation, a later date should be fixed up.

While her father was away, Sheila had another violent attack of the abdominal pains. She came to me seeking immediate relief and further treatment.

I expressed my unwillingness to take up the case, telling her that the appendix was believed to serve no useful function in the body, and the operation involved no risk.

The gentleman who had accompanied her said, "Yes, we are definitely going to have the appendix removed. But the operation is to take place after several days, and she is having severe pains. We felt that it would be better if meanwhile she can be given some treatment for relieving the pain."

I advised her to start fasting immediately. I instructed her to take four or five drinks of warm water in a day. Among other measures, I advised hot and cold applications on the abdomen, as well as applications of wet clay. There was some amelioration of the pain. From the fourth day, hot and cold hip-baths were also started. The abdominal pain was cured within a week.

After eight days of fasting, she was put on liquid diet.

In the meanwhile, Sheila's father had returned. Sheila had such remarkable relief from the pains that everyone in the family was in two minds whether to proceed with the scheduled operation or not. After plenty of discussion, it was decided to consult the surgeon again. As the symptoms had disappeared entirely, and even pressure on the relevant areas of the abdomen did not cause any pain, he took another radiograph and carried out other investigations. The reports were so favourable that the surgeon declared the operation to be no longer necessary.

10. MALARIA

Devkiprasad Pandey, a Mumbai businessman dealing in tea, had been to Assam on business about a year ago. Around the bungalow where he had put up, there was dense and luxuriant vegetation, and there was a small pond nearby. He was charmed by the pleasant atmosphere and beautiful natural scenery. But there were hordes of mosquitoes around. He could not sleep at night. In the mornings, he would feel tired and lethargic. Throughout his stay of one week there, this was his unvarying experience. He contracted fever even during his stay there. He returned to Bombay as soon as the fever yielded to treatment with tablets. But the fever recurred in Bombay too.

His doctor diagnosed malaria and prescribed medicines. Devkiprasad was a busy man, and could not take the medicines at the appropriate times. After a few days there was a relapse. This time the symptoms were even more severe. He would shiver with extreme cold before the temperature would rise. Severe headache would accompany the rise of temperature. Occasionally he would vomit. The orthodox treatment was resumed. The severity of the attacks decreased a little. But the fever assumed a recurrent periodic form, with the attacks occuring regularly on alternate days.

Devkiprasad went from doctor to doctor, and consulted Vaidyas and Hakeems, too. Some treatments would prove fairly efficacious and he would feel better for a few days. But then the cycle of events would start repeating itself.

One day a mutual acquaintance brought him to me. His body was emaciated and his face pale. The eyes were popping out of their sockets. He coughed intermittently. On examination I found that his spleen had become considerably enlarged and the surface area of the abdomen over the spleen had become oversensitive.

Realising the gravity of the situation, I advised him to get himself admitted to a hospital and commence the established course of treatment. But Devkiprasad was fed up with medicines and was not prepared to try them all over again. He insisted now on being given Naturopathic treatment.

I recommended fasting. As a preliminary step, he was put on liquid diet for five days, during which he was given fruit juices, uncooked juices of raw vegetables, and soups of leafy vegetables. Other measures taken were steambaths and abdominal packs, with enemas given every third day. These measures effected considerable reduction in the severity of his headaches.

The fasts began in real earnest on the sixth day. Four or five drinks of warm water in a day, with sips of cool water permitted only if feeling really thirsty in between, were prescribed. He was allowed to take the juice of half a lemon, or two spoonfuls of orange or *mosambi* juice with water twice a day, if he felt so inclined.

In only four days the severity of the fever showed notable reduction. The cough had almost disappeared. He himself felt much more energetic than before.

The attacks of fever ceased from the eighth day. Though he had lost as much as 5 kilogrammes in this short period, I advised him to continue the fasts for some time.

On the twelfth day he complained of nausea, giddiness and a feeling of oppression. His breathing was quick and shallow, and his pulse erratic. This was followed by copious vomiting, through which a large quantity of noxious materials were discharged. I decided that this was the proper time to terminate the fast. There had been no sign of the fever for the previous four days. I put him on fruit and vegetable juices again. By bed time all his afflictions had melted away. His breathing was normal and his pulse regular.

After two days of liquid diet, he was allowed to start taking a little solid food. By gradual changes in the type and amount of solid foods permitted, he was led step by step to a normal diet. I advised him to keep to simple foods as a precautionary measure, and to fast for one day in a week.

When I met him two months later, he was in a glowing mood. Gratefully shaking hands with me, he informed me that he had had no fever after the treatment, and was feeling extremely well.

11. PERSISTENT FEVER

A few years back, a young man about 23 or 24 years of age came to me. He used to have attacks of fever every ten or twelve days. Temperature would shoot up to 102 – 103° F, and the fever would last for three days or so. It would yield to treatment, but could not be permanently shaken off. This had been going on for about two and a half years. Constant consumption of powerful toxic medicines had reduced his body to a skeleton.

He had taken a vast variety of medicines and injections. He had had radiographs taken, and blood, saliva etc. tested, as directed by various physicians. But all to no avail. Some doctor advised tonsillectomy. He promptly had his tonsils removed. But the fever persisted. No one was able to determine the real cause of the fever.

I declined to take up the case, as the cause of the disease was not ascertainable. How does one go about treating a patient without a proper diagnosis of his disease? But his entreaties continued.

At last I yielded and commenced treatment. I asked him to fast for two days, taking only water, and then subsist on liquid diet, taking enemas every two or three days. From the third day onwards, he was to take half a cup of bitter neem leaf juice, a glass of warmed orange or *mosambi* juice three times a day, and hot soups of leafy vegetables twice a day. If the fever recurred, he was to fast, taking nothing but water for the duration of the fever, and to resume his liquid diet when the temperature reverted to normal.

To his delighted surprise, the fever did not recur for twenty days. And when it did, it was like a parting salutation only. The temperature rose only to 100°F, and returned to normal the very next day. When he came to see me after six more months, he was glowing pink with health. "How are you now?" I asked him. "In excellent health, thank you, "he replied. "I have had no fever since then. At that time I was so emaciated that people presumed I was suffering from some terrible disease. No one was prepared to give his daughter to me in marriage. But—,"he smiled and produced an invitation card, "—the problem has now been solved. Please do attend the wedding ceremony."

12. CANCER

The troubles of George Smith, a resident of Kansas City in the USA, started when he was 51. A nodule developed on his neck just below the left side of his jaw. It gradually increased in size and grew painful. The family physician assumed that George had some respiratory injection that had resulted in the enlargement of a lymph gland on the neck. But administration of antibiotics failed to reduce the size of the growth, or the pain. The opinion of a consulting physician was, therefore, sought. He, too, did not consider the matter to be serious, but to be on the safe side he advised a blood test and biopsy of the growth. The growth was diagnosed as a malignant cancerous tumour on the basis of the investigation.

Then began a series of various drastic and deadly measures. George was put on chemotherapy, but the tumour continued to grow. Radiotherapy was commenced after a few days. George's hair began to fall off and the skin began to be darkened, but the tumour was not controlled. It had grown to such an extent as to render even speaking and swallowing difficult. The cancer was spreading, and signs of this were evident on the lower jaw and the left cheek. The doctors finally decided to remove the tumour. George had been reduced to being just a silent spectator in this merry-go-round of tests and treatments. He gave his consent to the operation without taking time to think. The tumour and part of the jawbone were cut out. Now it was no longer possible to take food orally; so a rubber tube was introduced into the stomach through the neck. Fifteen days later he was informed that his cancer had been successfully extirpated, and he could henceforth live a normal life. With the assurance that the wounds caused by the operation would heal after a few dressings, he was discharged from the hospital.

But the wounds did not heal. On the contrary, they began to fester. But still under the impression that the healing would not take long, he consulted a plastic surgeon for removing the disfigurement caused by the excisions. The surgeon agreed to operate. Before the operation, a routine check up was carried out, including tests of the urine, blood and stools, as well as X-rays of the chest. During this check up, the sad fact came to light that the cancer had already spread to the lungs. There was now no question of undertaking the cosmetic plastic surgery. The doctors now entertained no hopes of George's survival.

But, for reasons beyond comprehension, George continued to live. He passed fourteen years in this condition, unable to speak, and taking nutrition through the rubber tube. Often he contemplated suicide, but the thought of his wife prevented him from taking the final step.

One day, purely by accident, he came to hear about Dr. Wigmore and his treatment with sprouted, or germinated, wheat. Like a drowning man clutching at a straw, he decided to try this treatment. He went and saw Dr. Wigmore. His face was a hideous sight at the time because of the disfigurement. Dr. Wigmore listened to the history of the case, and carried out a thorough examination. She was in two minds about taking up such a case. But ultimately Dr. Wigmore yielded to George's insistence and admitted him to the hospital. The very next day he was started on wheat-sprout juice. On the first day, he was given four cups of the juice, one cup being given every three hours. But the next day, George contracted a cold and diarrhoea, and had a mild fever, too. Dr. Wigmore was alarmed. But George had made up his mind to stick to the system, for better or worse, sink or swim. Seeing his courage and determination, Dr. Wigmore continued the treatment.

The next day George was given the juice-diluted with a little water. This was repeated on the third day. In the evening of the third day the temperature returned to normal, and the diarrhoea and the cold were no longer in evidence. At the same time, the first positive sign of improvement became apparent: the foul smell had stopped emanating from the cancerous tissues. Undiluted juice of the sprouts was resumed.

After eight days, applications of cloth wetted with the juice of sprouted wheat on the festering wounds on the neck and the face were commenced. This resulted in a complete cessation of pus formation in the wounds within a matter of 15 days.

At the end of the third week, a great deal of improvement could be seen. George had begun to speak a little. The sun of hope had begun to peep through the dark clouds of despair.

By the end of the fourth week, something had happened that would have been considered impossible. The wounds on the jaw and the neck had slowly begun to heal. It was not long before the healing was complete. George was now able to take some food orally.

His weight had also increased a little during this treatment. He had gained seven kilogrammes in seven weeks. There was no need for George to continue to stay in the hospital. He thanked Dr. Wigmore and took her leave.

Some days after going home, he underwent a complete medical check up of the whole body by the most modern methods. There was no trace of cancer cells. The doctors were wonderstruck. They could not trust their eyes; but the facts could not be ignored. When George reported this news to Dr. Wigmore on the phone, she too was astonished.

When George met Dr. Wigmore after a few months, he had altered beyond recognition. He had undergone plastic surgery to remove the disfigurement caused by his disease – and by the treatment. He informed Dr. Wigmore that he was at the time getting his old house in Pennsylvania repaired, and was busy planning his future life.

He had acquired renewed self-confidence and a sanguine expectation of long years of healthy life ahead of him.

☆☆☆

Published by Navneet Publications (India) Ltd., Dantali, Gujarat.
Printed by Ambika Mudranalay, Ahmedabad – 380 004.

[3 – 7 – 2008 (15) : 4]